Strength Training for Beginners

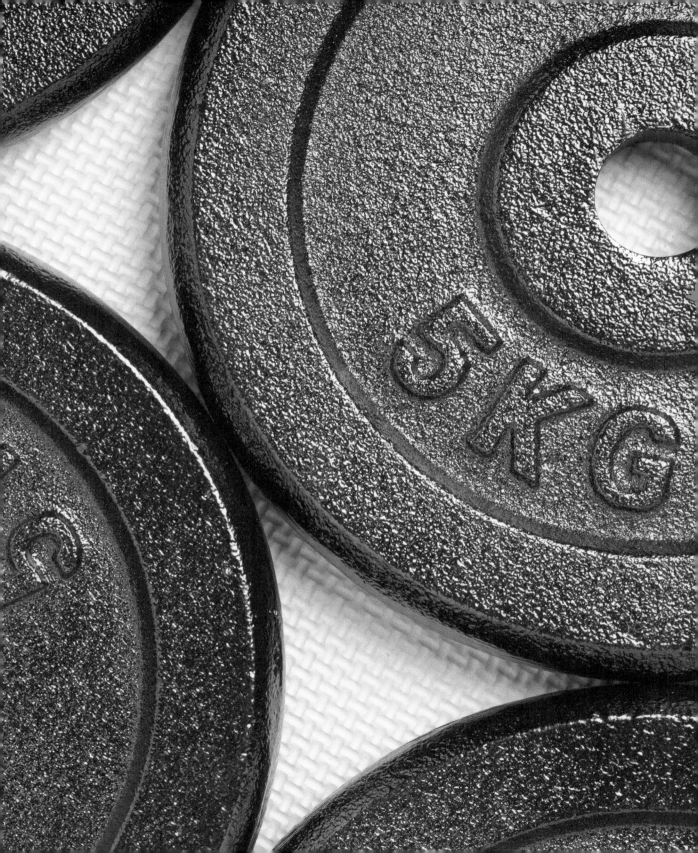

Strength Training for Beginners

A 12-WEEK PROGRAM TO GET LEAN AND HEALTHY AT HOME

KYLE HUNT

Illustrations by James Pop

ROCKRIDGE
PRESS

Interior and Cover Designer: Julie Schrader
Art Producer: Megan Baggott
Editor: Natasha Yglesias

ISBN: Print 978-1-64611-782-6 | eBook 978-1-64611-783-3
R0

To my unborn twins, Kyle Jr. and Eleanor.
I can't wait to meet you!

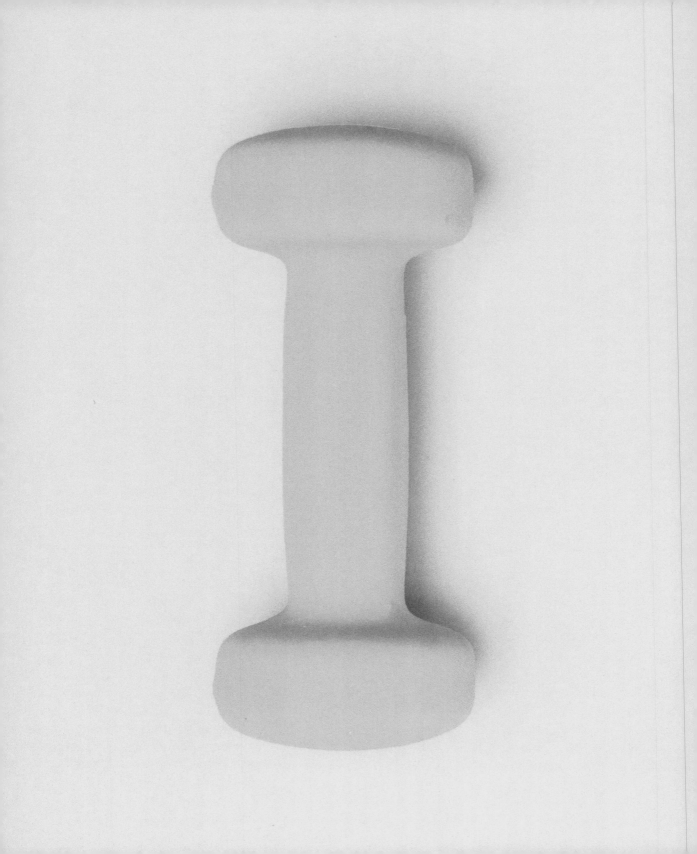

Contents

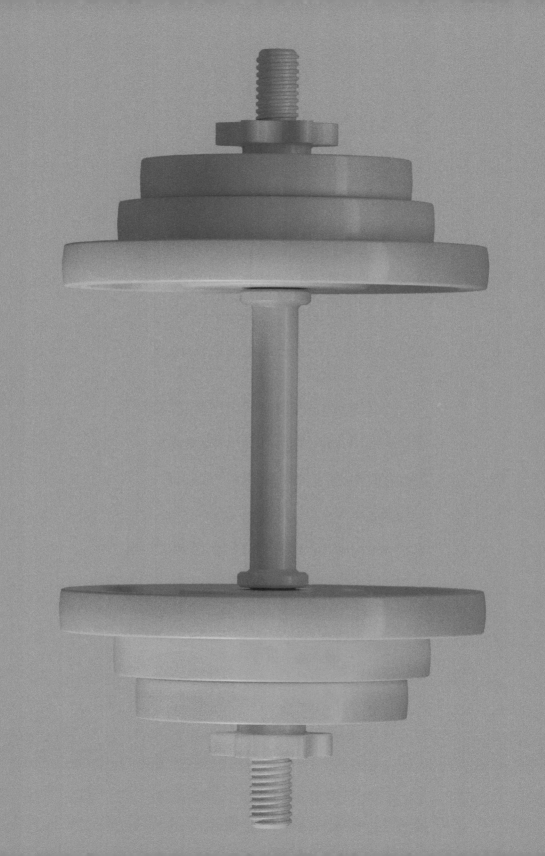

Introduction

Welcome to *Strength Training for Beginners*! I want to congratulate you for picking up this book. This is the first step in committing to your health and living powerfully for decades to come. The first step is often the hardest. My goal is to meet you where you are, since everyone begins their journey in a different place.

My fascination with strength started in my sixth-grade gym class. I was a tiny kid, easily one of the smallest in my grade. Having never worked out before, I wasn't sure what to expect when our class found out we would be spending the next few weeks in the weight room. I remember feeling nervous. Little did I know those weeks would have a huge impact on the rest of my life.

That class sparked a fire that continued through my teenage years. I started taking training seriously when I made the varsity wrestling team as an eighth grader. Being the smallest kid on the team, I knew lifting weights and getting stronger was going to help me level up. In high school, I was not only obsessed with lifting weights, but also with learning everything I could about the topic. As I grew older, I knew I wanted to make it part of my career. I became fascinated with the process, effects, and overall lifestyle that strength training had brought into my life and I wanted to help others achieve these same passions. Eventually, I earned a degree in exercise science and started my fitness company, Hunt Fitness.

Over the past ten years, I've worked with hundreds of people just like you. I believe one of the best ways to change your life is to change your body, and I've seen some amazing transformations. We get only one body to carry us through this life, so it makes sense to make it stronger and more resilient.

I wanted this to be an all-inclusive program. You don't need fancy equipment to get started. As you progress, new exercises will be introduced to help you along the way. There's practically an unlimited combination of ways to customize the program for your goals. I'll provide you with the information you need to make the necessary assessments and regulate your workouts based on your changing needs.

For beginners, learning proper technique is often a struggle, so I include in-depth descriptions along with images on how to perform every exercise discussed. Later, we'll look at a few tips and common mistakes to avoid. This book and its 12-week program are the beginning of your lifelong journey for strength. Let's get started!

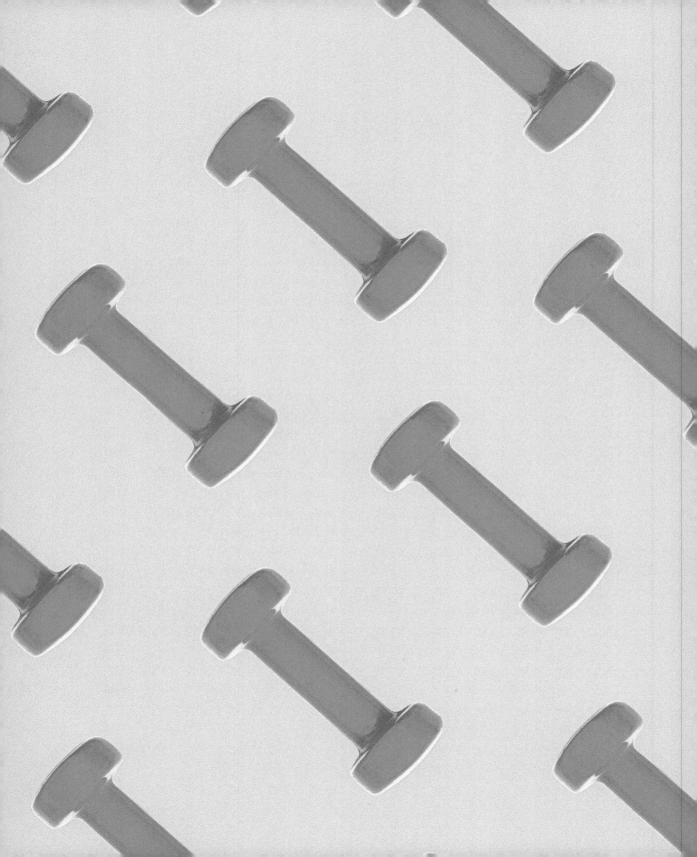

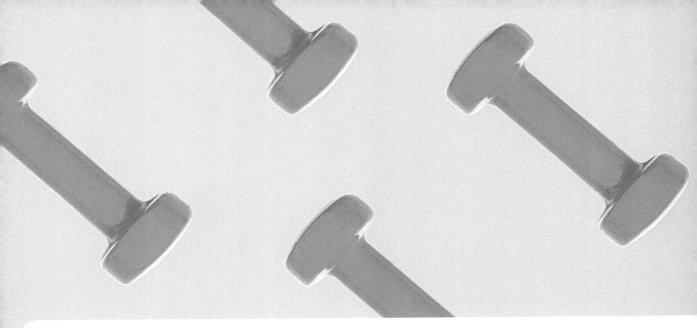

Part One

UNLOCK YOUR POWER

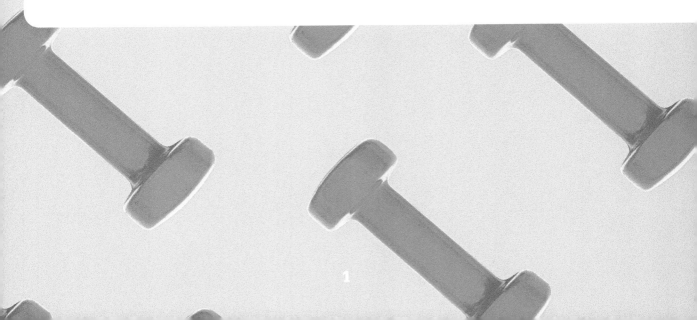

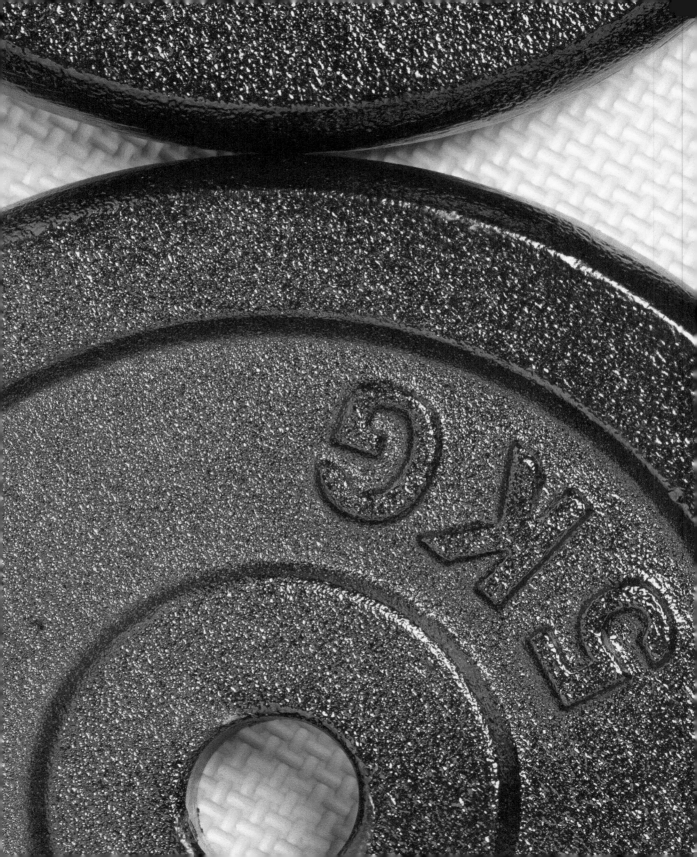

Chapter One

Getting Stronger

Strength training is a versatile form of exercise that can be beneficial for everyone as well as an activity that can be done over a lifetime. Aside from building muscle, a well-structured strength training program can help lower body fat, improve bone health, and boost cardiovascular health. This form of exercise can be structured to meet the needs of everyone, including novices, older folks looking for ways to improve their health and pursue longevity, and even current and former athletes who want to incorporate a new style of training into their existing routines.

While you probably imagine heavy barbells and big machines when thinking of strength training, that's only one way to do things. None of that is required for results. In fact, you can achieve a great workout by utilizing just your bodyweight and dumbbells. You'll also find that it is easy to transition to more advanced methods and modalities as you progress in your fitness journey.

How Training Works

The science of strength training and how muscles are built can best be described as a three-step process of stimulus, recovery, and adaptation.

The process starts in the gym with a **stimulus**, or a workout. Immediately after the workout, the body's **recovery** systems begin to heal and rebuild the tissue damaged by the workout. Although lifting weights sets the stage to make progress, you don't actually build muscle or gain strength while training. Muscle size and strength are actually both reduced immediately following a training session as the body repairs itself.

After a strength training workout, it's common to feel muscle soreness for 24 to 48 hours. This is called **delayed onset muscle soreness**, or **DOMS** for short. This happens while your muscles heal. Once the recovery occurs, so does the desired **adaptation**, or results. This is why it's important to take rest days for recovery and not push your body past its limits.

Bone and Muscle Health

In both the short and long term, lifting weights will improve muscular strength, increase muscle mass, and improve your ability to perform daily tasks. Overall, this makes you healthier and more resilient. These results, or adaptations, are easy to understand because we feel the muscles contracting and getting stronger. However, lifting weights strengthens more than just our muscles.

As we age, we lose bone density. Bones become more fragile and vulnerable to fracture and are more prone to breaking after even a minor fall. Physical activity, particularly lifting weights, offers the mechanical stimuli important for the preservation and improvement of bone health. As we age, the benefits of resistance training may result in further benefits, like a reduced risk of falls and injuries.

Muscle mass naturally diminishes with age as well. As muscle mass declines, so does our metabolic rate. This means it takes fewer calories to maintain bodyweight, and fewer calories to gain weight, too. As we age, lifting weights can be an important part in maintaining a healthy body composition and combating some of these natural struggles.

Balance and Mobility

Our bodies are designed to be able to move through full ranges of motion. When my daughter was a toddler, she would reach down to pick up a toy with her back flat, chest up, and hips sunk down into a perfect squat. Her form was better than most elite athletes! However, over time, day-to-day life slowly deteriorates our ability to move through ranges of possible motion unrestricted.

When I first started strength training, no one was talking about **mobility**, but in recent years the quality of movement has gained a lot of attention in the field. Exposing people to a variety of exercises sheds light on the inefficiencies in movement quality and a person's flexibility. Typically, people don't think about mobility until there is an issue such as pain, range of motion loss, etc. The truth is, improving movement through proper strength training can help prevent injuries and optimize performance.

Unlike running or biking, which are activities that create a lot of muscular imbalances if done exclusively, a quality strength training routine has the ability to distribute resistance equally throughout the entire body. This leads to a well-rounded muscular system more resilient to injury from muscular imbalances and overuse.

Live Long and Prosper

With strength training, it's easy to only think primarily about short-term benefits. This is especially true for younger folks. However, muscle mass has been shown to be a better predictor of mortality than simply looking at body mass index or bodyweight. To put it simply, the more muscle you have as you age, the lower your risk of death. Since muscle loss is a natural part of aging, the more muscle mass you build earlier in life, the more you're able to withstand losing. Many become less functional as they age, but strength training helps maintain the ability to perform daily tasks unlike anything else. Last but not least, the accumulation of muscle tissue helps keep the metabolism strong, which can help prevent the unwanted accumulation of body fat. Loss of muscle mass and strength have also been associated with an increased risk of dementia.

Instead of searching for the fountain of youth, Ponce de León should have just started working out!

Top 8 Strength Training Myths

1. **Strength training will make you bulky:** I wish this myth were true! The truth is, it's incredibly difficult to build enough muscle to look "bulky." The muscle-building process takes time and requires consistent training. Getting "too big" isn't something that will sneak up on you overnight, so it's not something you really need to worry about.

2. **Weightlifting is bad for the joints:** Any exercise can be dangerous if done incorrectly. Lifting weights with proper form and an appropriate weight is perfectly safe on the joints. When done properly, lifting weights can improve joint mobility and stability, leading to long-term joint health.

3. **You can Crunch or Sit-Up your way to a visible six-pack:** One of the biggest myths in fitness is the topic of spot reduction. Unfortunately, you cannot lose fat from one specific area of the body by performing exercises for that body part. While it's true that crunches help develop abdominal muscles, in order to get a *visible* six-pack, your body fat has to be low enough for the abs to show.

4. **Muscle turns into fat once you stop lifting weights:** This is a myth supported by examples of former strength trainers who gained weight after they stopped working out. It comes down to basic calories in versus calories out. If you continue eating more to support the extra calorie burn that strength training provides and then fail to dial it back when you stop, those extra calories will be stored as fat. Muscle and fat are different types of tissue and cannot turn into each other under any circumstances.

5. **You need to lift heavy weights to see results:** Lifting heavy weights is one way to make progress, but resistance is resistance. The body doesn't care if the added resistance is coming from a heavy barbell or just your bodyweight.

6. **Strength training makes you stiff and inflexible:** Can you believe there was a time when coaches prevented their athletes from lifting weights? The truth is, flexibility is only diminished immediately after lifting weights. There is no less flexibility once your body has recovered. In fact, strength training can actually improve flexibility.

7. **Strength training is difficult to learn:** The great thing about strength training is that it's highly versatile and meets you at your current ability level. You can take advantage of strength training by utilizing simple bodyweight exercises to start.

8. **You have to feel sore to make progress:** While soreness is sometimes part of the process, it's not always directly correlated *with* progress. You can have an effective workout even if you're not sore the next day.

Modern Science

When I bring other fitness experts on *The Absolute Strength Podcast*, one of my favorite questions to ask them is, "What have you changed your mind about lately?" This question is interesting because it digs into a fundamental aspect of science: New discoveries are happening, fast. If you're still doing everything the same as you were a few years ago, chances are those methods are already outdated. One area where research has changed over the last few years is the concept of training to failure.

When performing resistance training, going until you cannot complete any more repetitions (reps) is referred to as "training to failure." It was once thought that training to failure was essential to building muscle and gaining strength. Old-school lifters would even go as far as to say the only reps that matter are the last couple before you reach complete failure. But that's not necessarily the case. Over the past few years, research has shown there's not much of a difference between training to failure and stopping just shy of failure. However, a study in 2019 actually found greater adaptations in muscle growth from subjects who did not train to failure.[1] Regardless, the research is pretty clear: Training to failure is not nearly as important as it was once thought to be. Keep in mind this isn't an excuse to avoid hard workouts. Although research shows you can build muscle without going to the limit, you still have to make sure sets are challenging. I recommend stopping each set between 1 to 3 reps from failure. This ensures training is hard enough to facilitate progress but not so hard that it compromises proper form and limits recovery.

When it comes specifically to gaining strength, staying a few reps shy of failure is the way to go as well. Training to failure increases recovery time, compromises training frequency, and can lead to form breakdown. Strength is a skill, and like any skill, it gets better with high-quality practice. When gaining strength is the goal, training should be approached as "practice" as much as it is a workout. Each session is an opportunity to improve technique and increase your lifting skills, which will ultimately lead to your ability to demonstrate more strength.

---

1   Carroll, Kevin, Caleb Bazyler, Jake Bernards, Christopher Taber, Charles Stuart, Brad DeWeese, Kimitake Sato, and Michael Stone. "Skeletal Muscle Fiber Adaptations Following Resistance Training Using Repetition Maximums or Relative Intensity." *Sports* 7, no. 7 (July 11, 2019): 169. doi.org/10.3390/sports7070169.

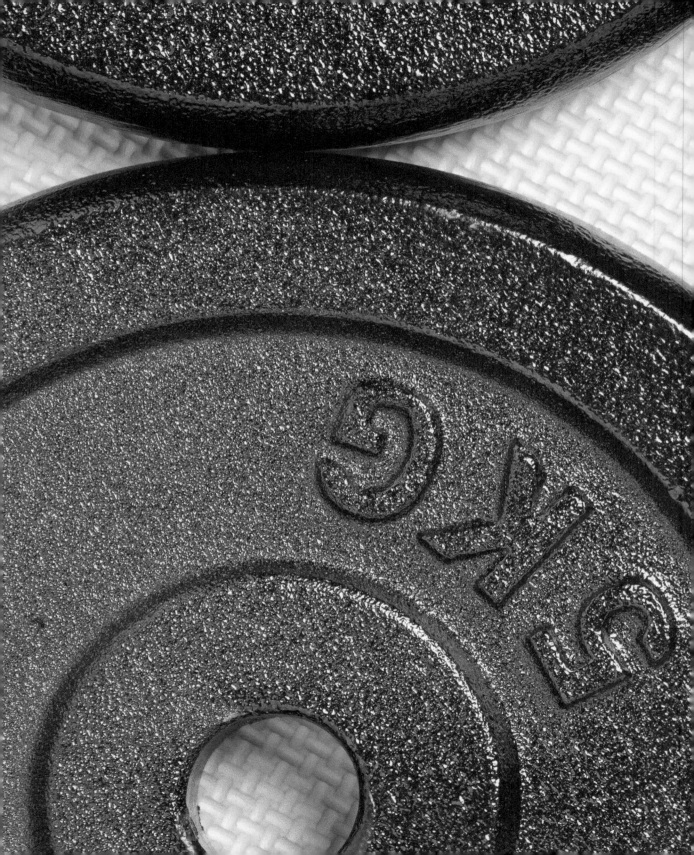

Chapter Two

Chapter Two

A Stronger Life

To be at your best in life and in the gym takes more than just hitting your workouts hard. Treating your body with good nutrition, recovery, sleep, and self-care will help take your results to the next level. The amount of progress made lifting weights is directly related to how well you're able to recover from your workouts. Over the years, I've found that this is often the missing link when results are lacking.

Nutrition

If you ask ten people what proper nutrition looks like, you'll probably get ten different answers. The truth is, nutrition doesn't have to be confusing. There's a difference between methods and principles. A quote from Harrington Emerson, an efficiency expert of the early 1900s, captures this perfectly: "As to methods, there may be a million and then some, but principles are few. The man who grasps principles can successfully select his own methods. The man who tries methods, ignoring principles, is sure to have trouble."

In this book, we're going to focus on the fundamental principles of nutrition, like eating mostly whole, unprocessed foods, consuming protein with each meal, eating lots of vegetables, consuming some fruit, and adding quality carbohydrates and fats as needed. We'll also talk about the necessity for proper hydration and how pre- and post-workout nutrition can improve performance and recovery.

FOOD AS FUEL

The food you eat has a direct correlation with how you look and feel, as well as how you perform in the gym. The good news is that you don't need to be overly strict with your nutrition to gain strength. Focus mostly on big-picture items. Eat three to four well-balanced meals per day, making sure to have a serving or two of protein at each, along with plenty of fruits and vegetables. Protein is arguably the most important macronutrient you need to build muscle and gain strength. Aim to consume around one gram of protein per pound of bodyweight. Add carbohydrates and fats as needed to support your energy demands. If you keep these basics in mind, you'll be off to a good start.

From the list on the following two pages, build each meal around one to two protein sources, depending on your bodyweight and protein needs, and be sure to include a serving of green vegetables. From there, add a serving or two of carbohydrates, depending on your bodyweight and energy demands. Finally, round the meal out with a serving of fat. This creates a well-balanced meal loaded with the right macronutrients, micronutrients, and fiber.

Quality Protein Sources (~20g of protein)

3 whole large eggs (also counts as a fat serving)

5 egg whites

3 ounces chicken breast

3 ounces turkey breast

3 ounces white fish (cod, haddock, tilapia, grouper, etc.)

3 ounces salmon (also counts as a fat source)

3 ounces pork loin

3 ounces lean red meat (sirloin steak or 95 percent lean ground beef)

1 cup low-fat Greek yogurt

1 cup low-fat cottage cheese

2½ cups low-fat milk

6 ounces tofu

1 scoop protein powder

Quality Carbohydrate Sources (~30g of carbohydrate)

½ cup oatmeal

⅔ cup rice

1 cup quinoa

2 slices whole-grain bread

1 whole-grain English muffin

3 rice cakes

6 ounces potatoes

1 medium apple

1 medium orange

1 medium banana

2 cups berries (blueberries, strawberries, raspberries, etc.)

2 cups carrots

Note: Green veggies such as broccoli, spinach, salad greens, peppers, asparagus, cucumbers, etc., are technically carbohydrates. However, their carbohydrate count is really low and consists mostly of fiber. Within reason, the more green veggies you eat, the better. Aim to have around a cup of green veggies at each meal.

Quality Fat Sources (~15g of fat)

2 tablespoons peanut or almond butter

¾ whole avocado

1 ounce almonds

1 tablespoon butter

1 ounce walnuts

1 tablespoon olive oil

1 ounce cashews

2 tablespoons salad dressing

1 ounce seeds (pumpkin or sunflower)

HYDRATION

When it comes to hydration, the body does a pretty good job of regulating fluid intake by adjusting our levels of thirst. The key is to have fluids readily available throughout the day. Water is best, but other drinks such as calorie-free flavored drinks, juice, milk, coffee, or tea work as well.

BEFORE THE WORKOUT

Pre-workout nutrition is very important. We want to make sure we're consuming food that will provide energy for the workout while also not causing indigestion, heartburn, or other digestive issues. Nothing is worse than being in the middle of a workout with a stomachache.

3 hours to 30 minutes before the workout

During this period, have a balanced meal consisting mostly of protein and carbo-hydrates. Having a serving of fat is fine as long as it sits well with your stomach. I recommend avoiding high-fiber foods in the pre-workout meal, so this is one meal where you can skip the green veggies.

Here are a couple of examples of solid pre-workout meals:

Example #1: 1 cup flavored low-fat Greek yogurt, 1 medium apple, 1 ounce almonds.

Example #2: 3 whole eggs, ½ cup oatmeal, a handful of blueberries.

Example #3: 1 scoop of protein powder, 1 medium banana, 1 to 2 tablespoons peanut butter

30 to 15 minutes before the workout

Immediately before the workout you should focus on being well hydrated. Make sure to drink 12 to 16 ounces of water 15 to 30 minutes before the workout. Try to accomplish this by drinking a bottle of water on your way to the gym.

Caffeine is one of the most widely used dietary supplements among fitness enthusiasts. This is optional, but consuming 100 to 300mg of caffeine pre-workout has been shown to have numerous benefits. Caffeine can reduce fatigue and increase strength during resistance training. This can be accomplished by having a cup of coffee, a sugar-free energy drink, or a pre-workout supplement.

AFTER THE WORKOUT

The need for a specific macronutrient breakdown post-workout has been overvalued in the past. However, this doesn't mean it's unimportant. At the end of the day, how your body responds to and recovers from training largely has to do with your total daily calorie and macronutrient intake. Put another way, the quality of your nutrition habits throughout the entire day is more important than what you consume specifically post-workout.

With that being said, having a well-balanced, protein-rich meal after a workout is a great idea.

Example #1: 3 to 6 ounces chicken breast, 1 cup rice, 1 cup broccoli, 1 tablespoon butter.

Example #2: 3 ounces of beef jerky, 1 low-fat cheese stick, 2 flavored rice cakes, 1 medium apple, 1 to 2 tablespoons peanut or almond butter.

Example #3: Protein smoothie with 1 scoop protein powder, ½ cup blueberries, 1 medium banana, 8 ounces low-fat milk.

Sleep and Self-Care

Sleep is vital to our health and well-being. It's been shown that a lack of sleep decreases performance in the gym, reduces your ability to recover from workouts, and even impairs metabolic function. The abundance of technology at our fingertips can make getting to bed on time even more difficult. It's just too easy to watch an extra episode of your favorite show on Netflix or scroll through social media while lying in bed. If we want to get the most out of our workouts, we need to take sleep seriously. The old recommendation that your mom told you of needing eight hours of sleep is close to accurate; I recommend aiming for seven to nine hours per night.

Tips to improve sleep:

- Wake up and go to bed at the same time every day, even on the weekends.

- Avoid caffeine after 4 p.m. The half-life (how long it stays in your system) of caffeine is between 4 and 6 hours.

- Avoid drinking too much liquid, including alcohol, before bed. You don't want to wake up in the middle of the night to use the bathroom. Also, alcohol negatively affects sleep quality.

- If you're going to eat before bed, make it a small snack. Don't eat a large meal before going to bed because digesting food will interfere with the circadian rhythms needed to suppress bowels at night.

- Put a stop to all screens, including computers, smartphones, and TVs, and avoid artificial light an hour before bed. If this isn't possible, look into getting some blue light blocking glasses. You can get them on Amazon for around $18.

- Keep the bedroom cool (not cold). Turn the thermostat down at night and sleep with just a sheet in the summer.

Stress

Managing stress is one of the most underrated aspects of performing well in the gym. Training is a stressor, but so are family troubles, lack of sleep, and an increased school workload. It's important that a program takes these factors into consideration, and one way of doing that is through autoregulation. Autoregulation is the ability to change a training program based on your responses to different stressors in life. Some days you'll feel really good. On those days, push yourself hard. But there will also be days where you don't feel as physically or mentally up to it. On those days, it's okay to take an extra rest day, use less weight, or pick an easier exercise to perform.

Finding Your Squad

One way to take things to the next level is to surround yourself with the right people. This is true in life, in business, and in the gym. If you want to get stronger, seek out people who are currently stronger than you and train with them.

If you decide to go to a gym, pick a location with members who have similar goals as you. There are a wide range of gyms available, from fancy commercial gyms to "hardcore" warehouse-style facilities. Each setup attracts a different crowd.

Even if you train at home, it's still important to find someone, or a group of people, to work out with. Not only is the social aspect a great way to stay motivated and have fun, but also a workout buddy is a great way to hold yourself accountable!

Getting Aerobic

While you get some cardiovascular benefits from strength training alone, it makes sense to include cardiovascular work in your weekly routine. Improving cardiovascular fitness is great not only for heart health and longevity but also for improving recovery time from weightlifting.

So many of us live sedentary lives outside of the gym. If you work a desk job and come home to relax on the couch for the night, chances are your daily step count is really low, even after lifting weights. If you don't like the idea of adding in formal cardio, you can simply track your daily steps. There are several apps that make this easy, and step trackers are built in to most newer phone models. Tracking your steps is something I've emphasized with my clients in recent years. I recommend getting between 8,000 and 10,000 steps per day. This can be achieved by going for a couple of 10-minute walks throughout the day, parking farther away at the grocery store, or playing a little extra with your kids.

If you would rather add in formal cardio sessions, try adding 30 minutes of low-intensity activity three to four days per week. This can be done by going outside for a bike ride or jumping on a treadmill, elliptical machine, Airdyne bike, or StairMaster. By keeping the intensity low, your cardio sessions will not negatively impact your strength training.

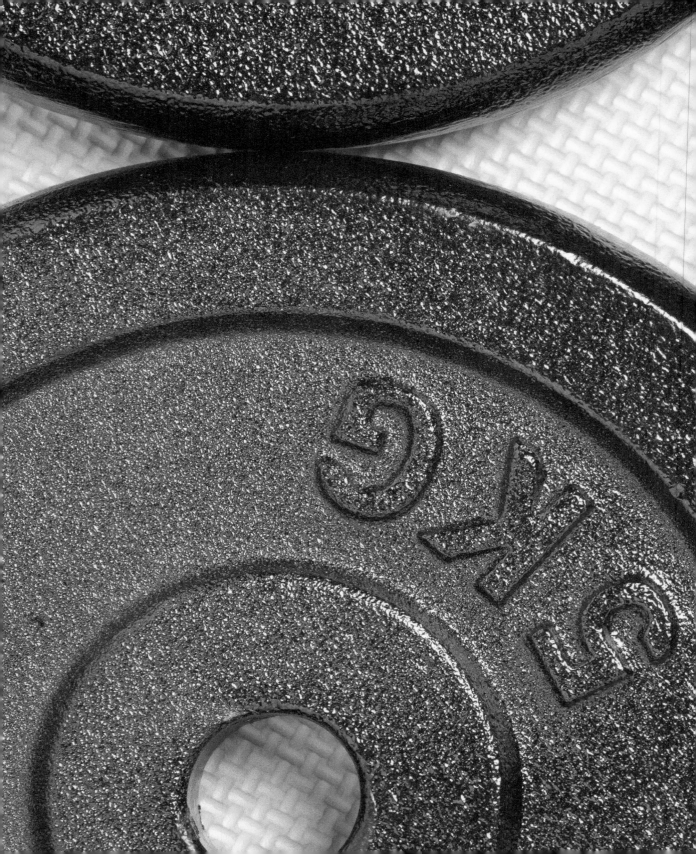

Chapter Three

About the Program

Now it's time to start training. In the following pages, I'll outline everything you need to know before jumping into the workouts, such as what equipment you need, how to progress in your strength training, and even what to do after you finish the 12-week program included. Read these sections carefully because a lot of this information will help optimize results in the short and long term.

Before we go further, it's important to point out that anyone who has not exercised for a while or who has health issues or concerns should consult with a doctor before starting a new exercise routine. Even if you've been exercising and don't have any health issues, if you haven't seen your doctor in the past year, it's a good idea to go in for a checkup.

Equipment Needs

The beauty of this program is that it can be started with little to no equipment. In month one, the program is bodyweight focused. For this part of the program all you need is a foam roller for the cooldown soft-tissue work and a doorway Pull-Up bar. You can pick both of those up on Amazon for between $20 and $50. If you want to hold off on buying any new equipment, you can repeat the bodyweight part of the program for additional months.

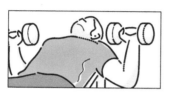

DUMBBELLS

Dumbbells typically get no love in strength training books, but they can be great tools to increase strength. In the second month of the program, I introduce dumbbells into the routine. For month two, the only new equipment you'll need is a set of dumbbells and an adjustable bench that has the capability to be flat or inclined.

Purchasing a dumbbell set can be expensive, but there are a couple of options to save money. The first is to look for used dumbbells. Unfortunately, a lot of people get excited and buy a bunch of fitness equipment before they've actually committed to using any of it. Their misfortune can be your gain. You can often find fitness equipment, specifically dumbbells, on Craigslist or at garage sales for a fraction of the in-store price.

Another option is to get a pair of adjustable dumbbells. These are dumbbells that have the capability to be multiple sets of weights all in one package. These are highly versatile and cost-effective. There are a few options within this category ranging in price, all of which will be more affordable than purchasing a full set of regular dumbbells.

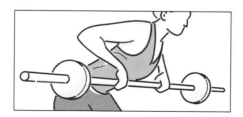

BARBELLS

In month three, the program combines bodyweight training, dumbbell training, and barbell training. Utilizing all three modalities is the best way to get stronger. In month three, you'll need a barbell, weight plates, and a squat stand or rack to complete the workouts. The fitness industry has seen a boom in production of at-home workout equipment in recent years. This has caused fitness equipment to become more available as well as more affordable. I recommend getting a 300-pound barbell set, which comes with a standard 45-pound Olympic barbell and weight plates equaling 300 pounds. This will be enough to get you started. Once you get strong enough to need more, you can buy additional weights individually. Deciding between a squat stand and a squat rack really comes down to price and space. If you have the extra money and space, I recommend going with the full squat rack, as this will allow you to do pretty much any barbell exercise in existence. The downside is that they take up a lot of space and can be pricy. For this program, you can get by with just a squat stand. Although not as versatile as a squat rack, it is more affordable and doesn't take up much space.

The Truth about Stretching

Static stretching and how it fits into a training program has been a lightning rod topic over the years. Static stretching is when you hold a stretch in a challenging position for a period of time. Back in the day, it was widely accepted to perform static stretching before gym class, playing a sport, or working out. However, recent research has shown the limitations of this style of stretching pre-exercise. This leads to people discounting the value of stretching altogether. As it turns out, stretching is best done at the end of the workout when the muscles are warm and the body is ready to unwind. Static stretching at the end of a workout has been shown to be a reliable way to increase flexibility and range of motion.

Coinciding with the elimination of static stretching during the warm-up period has been the rise of dynamic stretching. Dynamic stretching involves actively moving the muscles and joints through full ranges of motion. This has been shown to be a great addition to the warm-up.

You'll notice the 12-week training program takes advantage of dynamic stretching during the warm-up and static stretching in the cooldown. We use the dynamic movements to get the body ready to work out and the static stretches to improve flexibility and help speed up muscle recovery.

Post-Workout Stretches / Foam Rolling

Stretch #1: Couch Stretch

The Couch Stretch is a great movement to stretch the quads and hip flexors. It works great after a workout, but you can also do it on rest days if your legs or hips are tight. To do the Couch Stretch you'll need a bench, couch, or just a wall.

Place your lead leg in a lunged position, with the opposite knee touching the ground and the opposite foot elevated up on a bench. The back knee should be in a straight line with the front edge of the bench. Initiate the stretch by pressing your hip forward. Repeat on the opposite side.

Keep the rib cage down and core tight while performing this stretch! Avoid letting the lower back round.

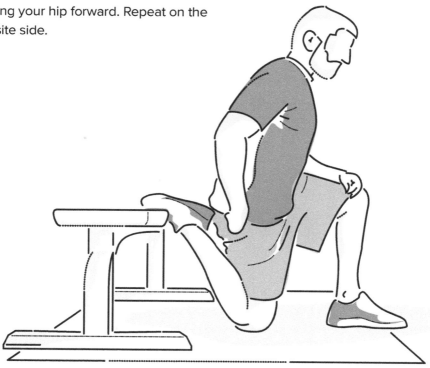

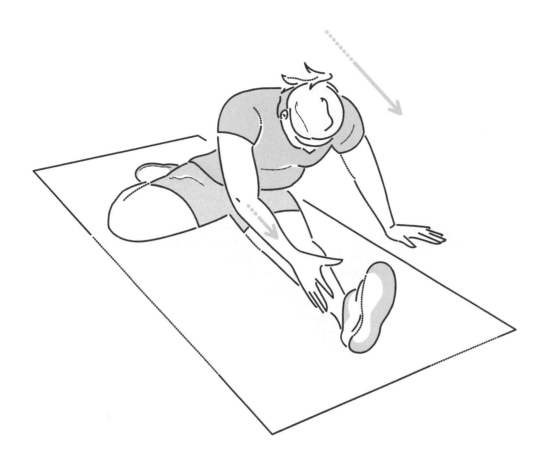

Stretch #2: Hurdle Stretch

The Hurdle Stretch has been a staple in physical education classes for years because of its ability to stretch the hamstrings and hip flexors. However, what many gym teachers got wrong was the timing. This stretch is best done after exercise, not before.

Get in a seated position and raise one knee 45 degrees from your hips. Position the other leg straight out in front of you. Reach along the straight leg as far as you can and hold. Repeat on the opposite side.

Don't cheat by bending the knee: Keep the extended leg as straight as possible.

Stretch #3: Lat Stretch

When you focus on building muscle and strength in the lats, the added strain can leave them tight and bunched up. This can cause poor overhead mobility, bad posture, and shoulder pain. The standing Lat Stretch is simple and easy to perform.

Stand facing a fixed bar or sturdy implement. Grab the bar or implement with two hands around waist height. Allow the hips to fall back while you bend over and lean your torso toward the stretched arms. Hold the stretch in this position.

A mistake people often make with the Lat Stretch is actually maintaining too much tension in the muscles. Make sure you relax the lats and allow them to fully stretch.

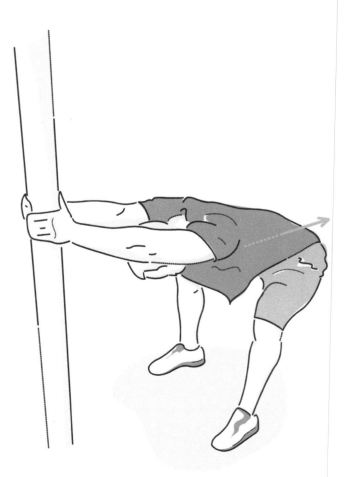

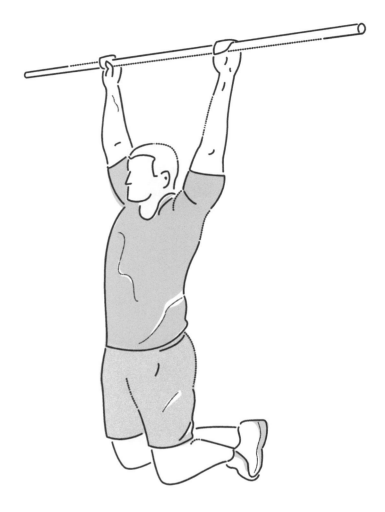

Stretch #4: Dead Hang

The Dead Hang is the simplest thing you can do to improve shoulder health and overhead positioning and decompress the spine all at the same time. Over time, it can help open up the shoulders and increase your range of motion. The limiting factor initially will be grip strength. Eventually your grip strength will catch up as a secondary benefit to improving your shoulder health.

Grab an overhead bar with an overhand grip about shoulder-width apart. Relax the whole body, making sure to reduce tension specifically in your shoulders and lower back. Keep your arms straight. Last but not least, just hang for the time duration (10 to 15 seconds).

Foam Roll Series #1: IT Band

It's very common for the IT band, which is located along the outside of your legs, to become tight and cause knee pain. A foam roller can help loosen up the area.

Lie on your side and place a foam roller under the outside of your leg. Slowly slide your body down the roller, moving from the hip to the knee until you find a tight spot. It's likely the entire IT band isn't tight, so the key is spending extra time in the areas that need attention. Repeat on the opposite side.

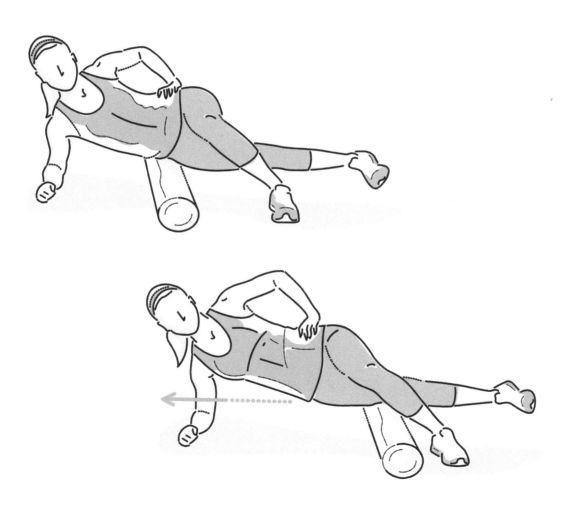

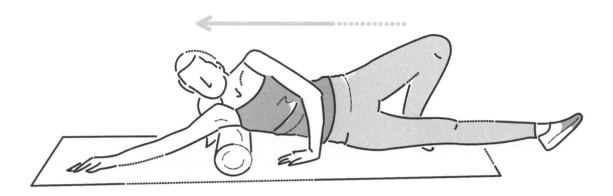

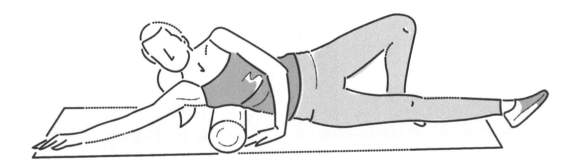

Foam Roll Series #2: Lats

The lat muscles are prone to getting tight and bunched up. This can negatively impact overhead positioning and ultimately lead to shoulder pain.

Lie on your side and position the foam roller underneath your armpit on your lat. Slowly slide your body down the roller until you encounter a tight spot. Hold the roller on the tight spot and move your arm in different overhead positions to help loosen the muscles. Repeat on the opposite side.

Foam Roll Series #3: Adductors

The adductors are the forgotten muscles of the lower body—until they are sore. Located on the inside of your thighs, they come into play during Squats and Deadlifts, among other lower body exercises.

Lying facedown, position the inside of your leg on a foam roller. Keeping the leg relaxed, slide the roller from the knee up to the groin area. When you roll onto a tight spot, create more pressure by driving your hip toward the ground. Repeat on the opposite side.

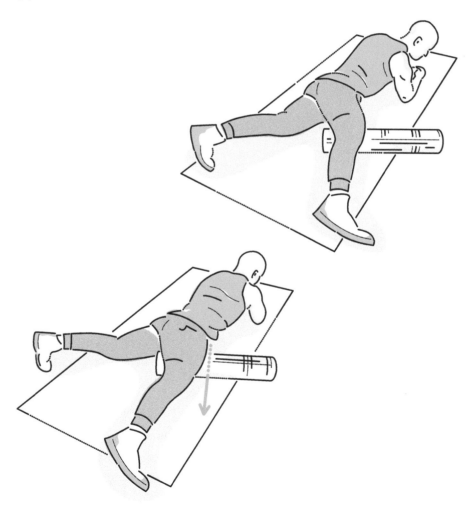

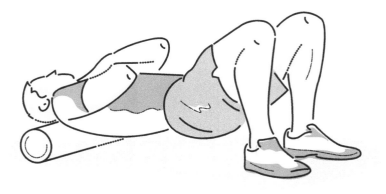

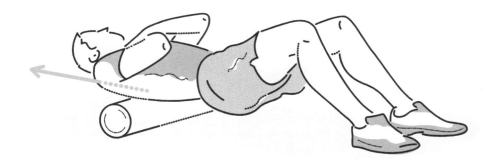

Foam Roll Series #4: Upper Back

Foam rolling your upper back is a great way to open up the entire thoracic region.

Lying faceup, wrap your arms around your chest and place the roller at the base of your rib cage. Slide your hips out and back to move your upper back across the roller. A common mistake people make with this movement is rolling back and forth aimlessly for a couple of seconds before finishing up. That doesn't do anything. Take your time, roll slowly, and when you find a tight area, spend extra time there. You can even arch your back a bit to dig in deeper.

Here Come Results

This 12-week program was designed as a complete strength training routine. With the inclusion of bodyweight, dumbbell, and barbell exercises, it attacks multiple strength modalities throughout the three months. Bodyweight exercises are great at improving the strength-to-bodyweight ratio, dumbbell exercises are great at training each side of the body equally and improving stabilization, and lastly, barbell training is the best method to improve maximal strength.

Every workout will include both lower and upper body exercises designed to work the full body each session. Although the workout program is only three days per week, you can stay active on your rest days. This is a perfect time to go for a bike ride, take a yoga class, or play a round of golf. The key is to keep the off-day activity low intensity. Since I know some of you will be ambitious and think more training is better, I want to reiterate: That's not necessarily the case. Rest and recovery are important parts of the program. Don't try to do too much!

Neural adaptations primarily drive strength gains in the first 12 weeks, which means you can gain strength quickly just by getting more proficient at the exercises. This occurs before your body has even had the chance to build any muscle. Keep good notes of how each exercise feels, how many reps you do, and how much weight you use. You can use this information to "beat the logbook" and build in progression each week.

Moving on Up

After you finish the 12-week program, you have a couple of options. The first is simply to start back at the beginning and run through the 12-week program a second time. Since you'll be familiar with the movements and likely stronger than you were before, you should be able to perform better a second time. Feel free to do more reps, select more challenging exercises, or use heavier weights.

Another option is to repeat month three a second time. Since month three includes bodyweight, dumbbells, and barbells, it's the most well-rounded month and best suited to be repeated.

If you want to try something different entirely, check out one of my other books, *Bodybuilding for Beginners*. There, I focus more on building muscle. It would be a great complement to the 12-week strength building routine you just completed.

Additionally, after you finish the 12-week program you may want to add some new equipment to your home setup or look into joining a gym. As you progress in your fitness journey, having more tools at your disposal can help keep things fresh and interesting!

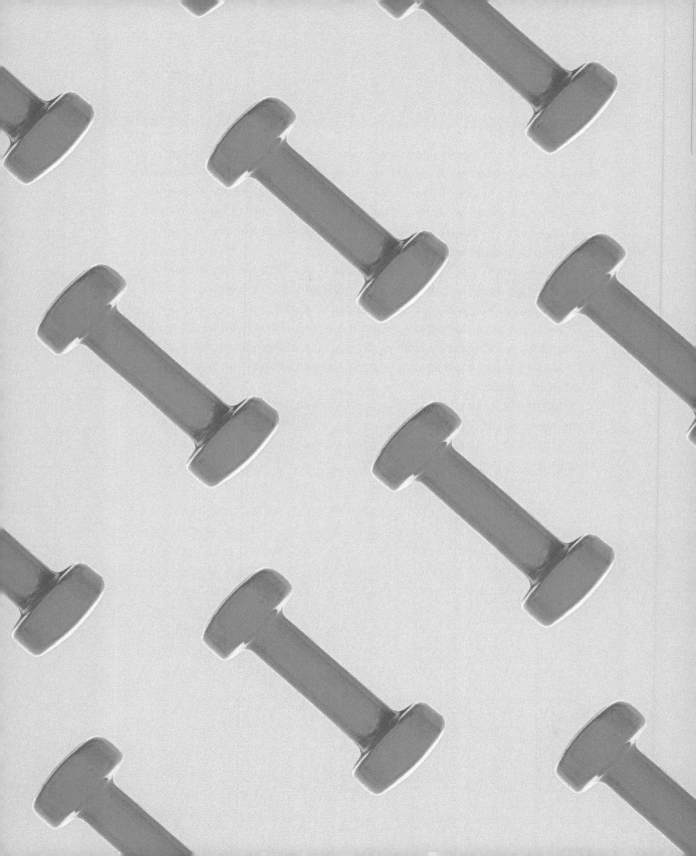

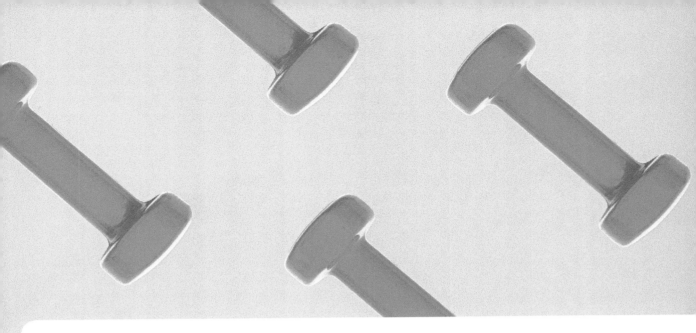

Part Two
THE EXERCISES

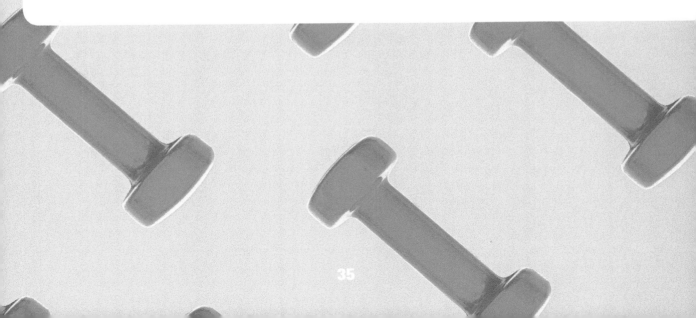

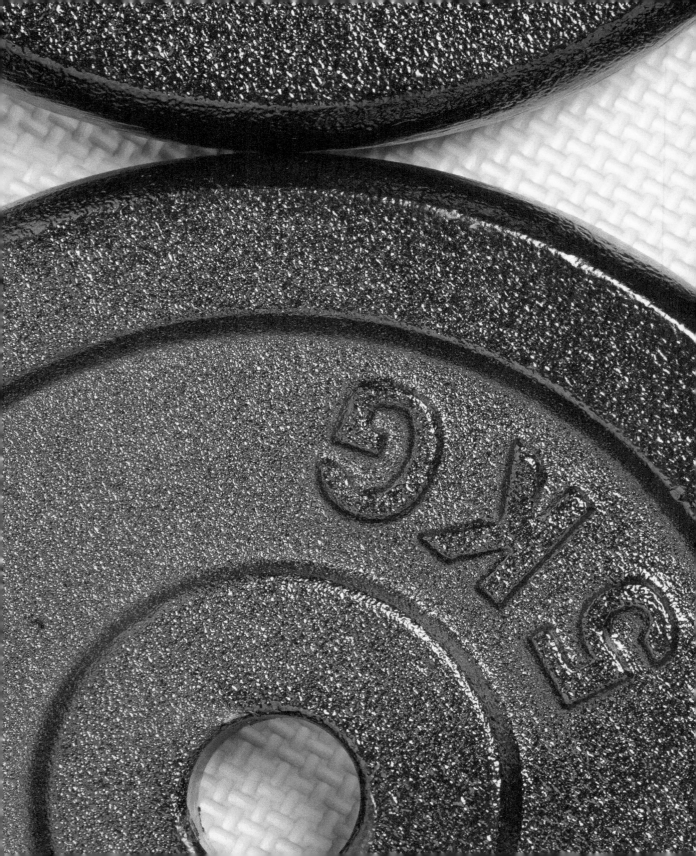

Chapter Four

Warm-Up Exercises

As with most things in the fitness industry, there's a lot of debate about how to warm up properly for a resistance training workout. The majority of people fall into two camps: the "old-school" approach of recommending very little or no warm-up at all, and those who spend 45 minutes to an hour warming up for a 15-minute workout. The best choice is somewhere in the middle.

Jumping Jacks

Specific Muscles Involved: Full Body

I love including Jumping Jacks in warm-ups because almost everyone has done them before, so there's not much, if any, learning curve. Jumping Jacks target your arms, legs, core, and shoulders all at once. All warm-ups would benefit from including Jumping Jacks!

Instructions

1. Stand straight with your legs shoulder-width apart and your arms at your sides.

2. Get into position, with the knees bent and core tight, and use your legs to jump up into the air.

3. As you jump, simultaneously extend your legs and arms out to the sides, creating an "X" with your body. Continue stretching your arms until they go over your head.

4. Return to your starting position and repeat for the desired amount of reps.

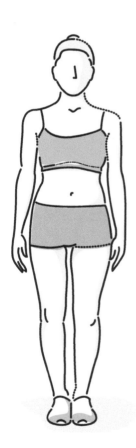

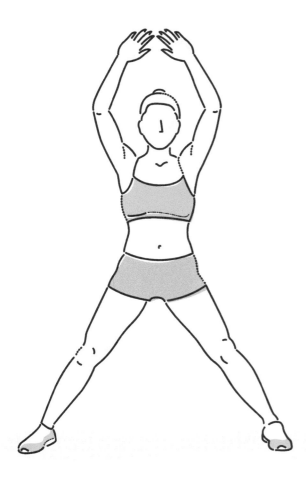

Practice Makes Perfect

Don't be out of sync! All the parts of your body should be in perfect harmony while you're performing this movement. Your arms and legs should be going out and coming in at the same time.

Training Tip

Use a full range of motion. Make sure you're bringing your legs out wider than shoulder-width apart and bringing your arms fully overhead on each rep. Don't shortchange the exercise by using a limited range of motion.

Easy Does It

Invisible Jump Rope: **An alternative to the Jumping Jack is what I call the Invisible Jump Rope. Stand in place and jump up and down while moving your hands like you are using a jump rope.**

Mountain Climbers

Specific Muscles Involved: Shoulders, Triceps, Core

The Mountain Climber is, in my opinion, a very underrated calisthenic. It activates a multitude of muscles and gets the heart rate up. Similar to the Jumping Jack, this is a basic exercise that's easy to learn. There are two major benefits of including the Mountain Climber in the warm-up: shoulder stability and core activation.

Instructions

1. Get into a Push-Up position, with your palms flat and a bit wider than shoulder-width apart. Make sure your weight is distributed evenly between hands and toes.

2. Your back should be flat, your core engaged, and your head in alignment with your spine.

3. Bring your right knee forward under your chest as far as you can. Then, in one motion, pull the right knee back (placing the right foot back on the ground) and bring the left knee in under your chest.

4. Keeping your hips level, continue that alternation by "running" your knees in and out while maintaining core control for the desired amount of reps.

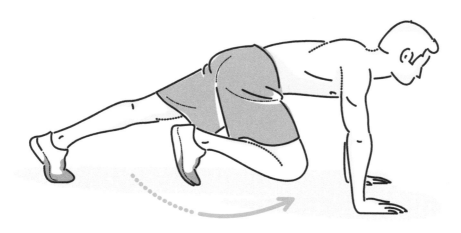

Practice Makes Perfect

Don't bounce on your toes. A common mistake with Mountain Climbers is to do this as you move. When you bring your knees up under your chest, keep your core engaged and your toes in contact with the ground.

Training Tip

It's not a race. Mountain Climbers can be done with a fast pace for a cardiovascular workout. For our purposes, however, we want to go slow and move through a full range of motion in order to get our shoulders, arms, and core ready to work out.

Easy Does It

Instead of starting in a Push-Up position on the floor, you can elevate your hands up on a bench. This allows you to perform the movement without supporting as much of your bodyweight with your hands. Other than the different hand placement, perform the exercise the same way.

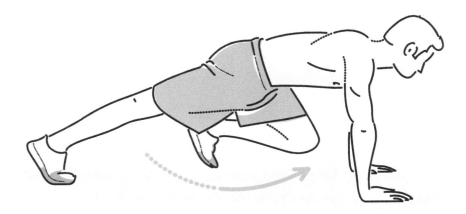

Arm Circles

Specific Muscles Involved: Shoulders, Arms, Upper Back

Arm Circles may offer the biggest benefit-to-effort ratio of any exercise in this book. Doing a few Arm Circles as part of your warm-up won't turn you into The Hulk, but it can help prevent injuries and get your shoulders ready for heavy pressing!

Instructions

1. Stand with your feet shoulder-width apart. Extend your arms parallel to the floor to form a "T".

2. Circle your arms forward using small, controlled motions, gradually making the circles bigger until you reach a full range of motion.

3. Reverse the direction of the circles after completing the desired amount of reps following the steps above.

Practice Makes Perfect

Stay in control! Keep your arms tense and controlled to avoid using momentum.

Training Tip

Keep your core braced like you are getting ready to take a punch.

Easy Does It

Bent-Elbow Arm Circles: To make the movement easier, bend your elbows 90 degrees and perform the movement from that position.

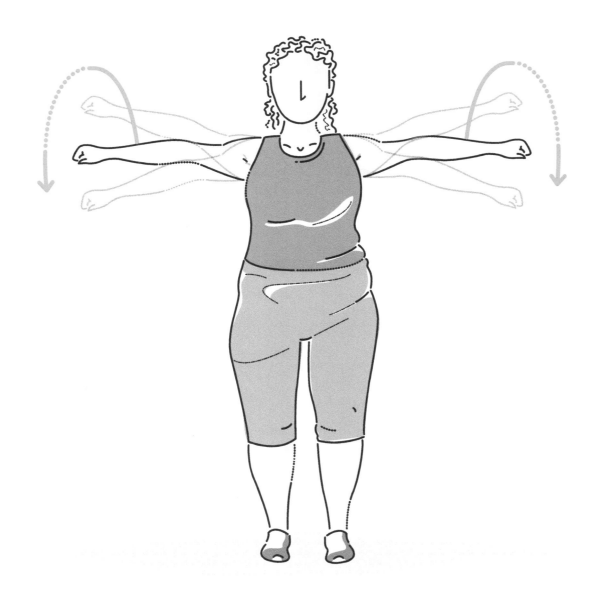

Scapular Push-Up

Specific Muscles Involved: Shoulders, Upper Back

Maintaining proper function and mobility of the scapula (shoulder blade) is important for all upper body strength movements. The problem is that doing a lot of heavy pressing—like the Bench Press (see page 134) and Overhead Press (see page 142)—can cause scapular mobility issues. The Scapular Push-Up is a simple solution to the problem.

Instructions

1. Start in a Push-Up position with your hands directly underneath your shoulders and your toes touching the floor.

2. Keep your body in a straight line and your head relaxed in a neutral position, aligned with the rest of your spine. Tighten your core and glute muscles so your hips don't sink.

3. Keep your arms fully extended and retract (pinch together) and protract (spread apart) your shoulder blades, causing your chest to lower and raise slightly. The range of motion is small. All of the movement should take place in the shoulders.

Practice Makes Perfect

Keep it simple. The biggest issue people have with the Scapular Push-Up is bending the elbows to create an illusion of a greater range of motion. Keep the elbows locked out and only move the shoulder blades through retraction and protraction.

Training Tip

Pause at the bottom and the top of the rep to help "feel" the stretch.

Easy Does It

To make the movement easier, you can do these on the floor from the knees instead of the feet.

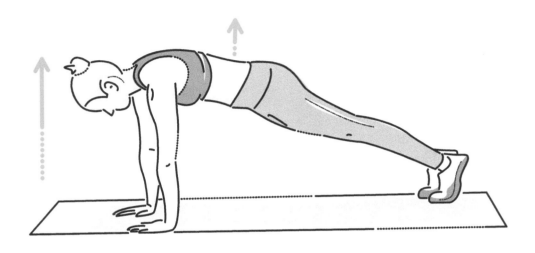

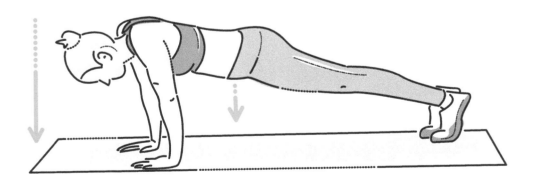

Bird Dog

Specific Muscles Involved: Core, Lower Back

The Bird Dog is an excellent exercise for core stability and lower back health! If you have reoccurring lower back pain, this is a great exercise for you to do on rest days as well as in the warm-up.

Instructions

1. Kneel on the floor on all fours (quadruped position) with knees hip-width apart, your hands shoulder-width apart, your core tight, and your back in a neutral alignment.

2. Without letting any movement occur in the lower back, extend one leg backward while simultaneously raising the opposite arm out in front until both extremities are fully extended.

3. Hold the extended position for a few seconds then return your hands and knees to the starting position.

4. Repeat on the opposite side.

Practice Makes Perfect

Don't let the lower back round or sag. Keep the core braced and the spine neutral at all times.

Training Tip

At the start of this movement, tighten the core, upper back, shoulders, and glutes as much as possible. The greater the tension you generate, the more beneficial the exercise is.

Easy Does It

Half Bird Dog: If you have difficulty with the Bird Dog, begin by just extending one leg at a time and not extending the arms.

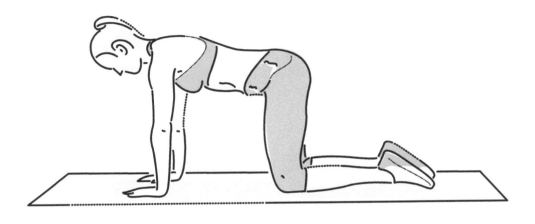

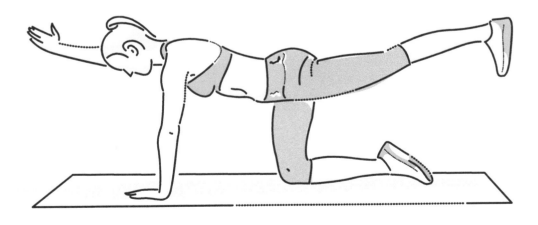

Leg Swings

Specific Muscles Involved: Quadriceps, Hamstrings, Glutes, Hips

Leg Swings are dynamic warm-up exercises that prepare the lower body for activity. Unlike static stretches, dynamic stretches allow you to move through a range of motion. This not only reduces the chance of injury, but also helps improve performance on lower body exercises.

Instructions

1. Stand with feet shoulder-width apart and extend your arms in front of you against a wall or a sturdy object. There should be enough room for you to swing your legs in front of you.

2. Stand on your left leg and extend your right leg out to the side so that it's just off the ground.

3. Swing the right leg to the outside as far as you can, then swing it back toward your body, crossing the left leg, as far as you can. This completes one rep.

4. Finish the set and repeat on the opposite side.

Practice Makes Perfect

Avoid opening up your hips when swinging your leg out to the side. Keep your core tight and hips square throughout the entire movement.

Training Tip

Keep your legs loose. Try to take out all of the tension from your hips down.

Easy Does It

Front and Back Leg Swings: **You can also do Leg Swings front to back instead of, or in addition to, side to side.**

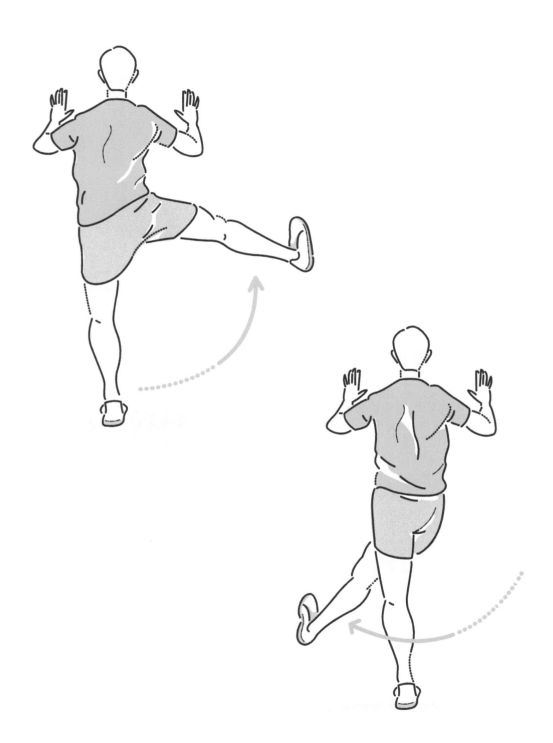

Thoracic Bridge

Specific Muscles Involved: Hips, Shoulders, Thoracic Spine

In today's society, so many of us spend a lot of time in front of computers or staring down at phones in hunched positions. Eventually, this hunched position leads to poor posture along with decreased hip, shoulder, and thoracic mobility, which reduces movement quality and makes it extremely hard to perform well in the gym. Luckily, the Thoracic Bridge addresses these issues! After adding this exercise into your warm-up, you'll immediately feel the benefit.

Instructions

1. Start in a quadruped position with the knees slightly off the ground and your hands shoulder-width apart. Your weight should be equally distributed between hands and toes.

2. Lift your right hand and left foot off the ground at the same time.

3. While bracing on the left arm, bring the left leg under your body through to the other side, rotating your hips out and placing both feet on the ground. At this point, your hips should be facing up at the ceiling and the chest toward the wall.

4. Once you get your hips rotated and both feet on the ground, reach your right arm across your body.

5. Finish the movement by extending your hips up toward the ceiling and holding for a few seconds.

6. Return to the starting position and repeat on the opposite side.

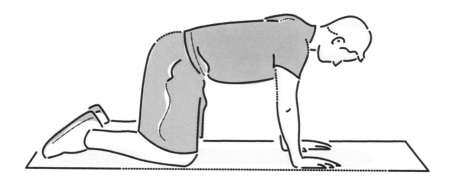

Practice Makes Perfect

Don't bend the elbow. A common mistake people make is bending the elbow on the bracing arm. We want to keep that arm as straight as possible to avoid losing shoulder stability.

Training Tip

Flex your glutes and try to drive your hips as high as you can at the top of the movement.

Easy Does It

The Standing Wall Touch: **An easier alternative to the Thoracic Bridge is the Standing Wall Touch. Stand about a foot in front of a wall, facing away from it. Reach back and touch the wall with both hands, rotating at the waist to the right. Hold the stretch for a couple of seconds before returning to the starting position and repeating on the left side.**

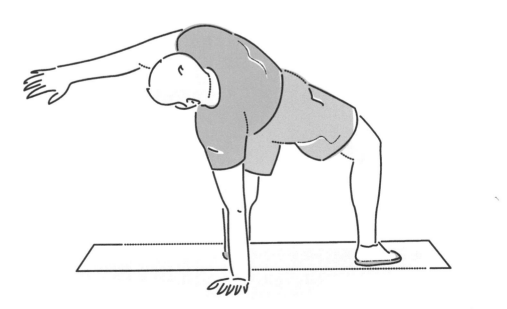

Fire Hydrant

Specific Muscles Involved: Glutes, Hips

After performing this movement, you'll probably be able to guess why people call it the Fire Hydrant. The Fire Hydrant is a great movement to help prepare your glutes and hips for the workout. Getting the glutes firing and the hips mobile is a wonderful way to prevent injuries from lower body exercises.

Instructions

1. Start in a quadruped position with your hands directly under your shoulders and your hips over your knees.

2. Keep your right knee at a 90-degree angle as you slowly raise your leg to the right until parallel to the ground. Hold this position for 5 to 10 seconds before lowering your leg back to the ground. Repeat on the opposite side.

Practice Makes Perfect

Don't rotate the torso. It's important to make sure you're opening your hip throughout the movement rather than rotating your torso to elevate your knee.

Training Tip

Flex your glute at the top of the movement.

Easy Does It

Standing Lateral Leg Raise: **An easy variation to the Fire Hydrant is a Standing Lateral Leg Raise. Standing straight, raise one foot off the ground and lift it laterally as far as you can. Bring the leg down slowly and repeat for the desired number of reps. Complete reps on both sides.**

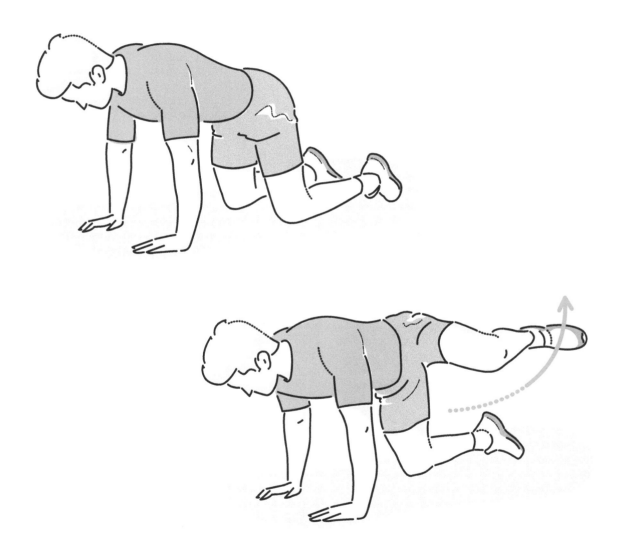

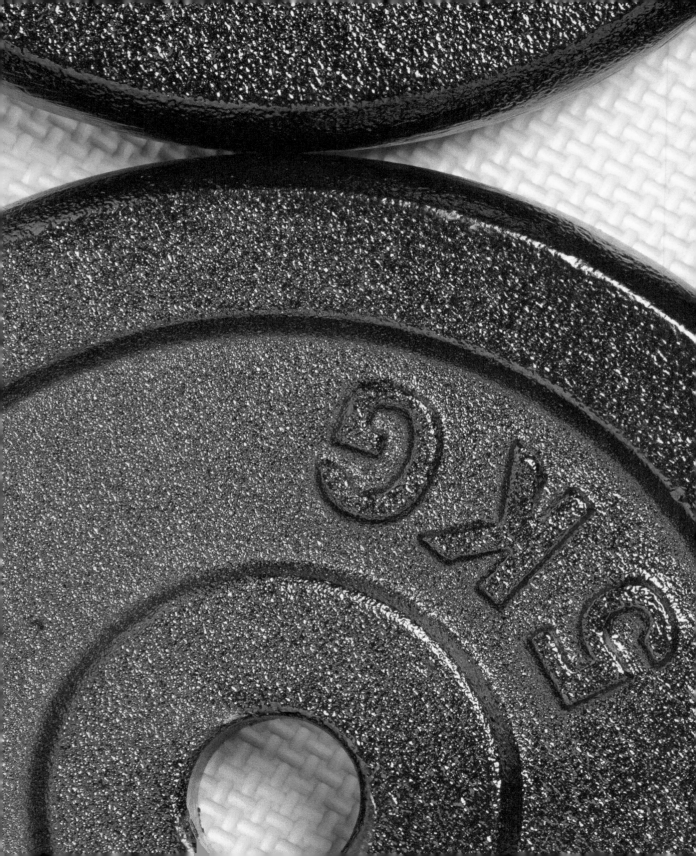

Chapter Five

Bodyweight Exercises

There are many different understandings of strength in exercise. Relative strength deals with strength-to-bodyweight ratio, and bodyweight training is one of the best ways to develop relative strength. Having high relative strength and being able to control your bodyweight is critical for excelling in athletics and daily life.

Another benefit of bodyweight training is that it's always there: You can get a quality workout anywhere and at any time.

One of the keys to successful bodyweight training is knowing and understanding **progressions** and **regressions**, or the ability to make the exercises harder or easier. To help you with this, each exercise in this section includes a more challenging option in addition to an easier one. This will allow you to more accurately pick the right exercise for your current strength and ability.

Push-Up

Specific Muscles Involved: Chest

The Push-Up is one of the most fundamental bodyweight exercises and can be a valuable tool for any training program. During a Push-Up, your hands and feet are fixed to the ground. As you lower yourself, your scapula is free to move, which is unique from almost any other chest exercise. Mastering the classic Push-Up is the first step to having a strong upper body.

Instructions

1. Get on the floor, facedown, and place your hands on the ground shoulder-width apart. Start with your arms fully extended and your legs straight. Your body should form a straight line, so keep your hips in line with your spine.

2. Lower yourself by bending the elbows until your chest almost touches the floor, making sure to keep your core engaged.

3. Once you reach the bottom, push up with your arms, lifting your upper body back to the starting position. Repeat for the desired amount of reps.

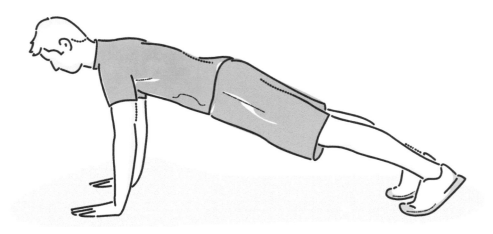

Practice Makes Perfect

A common mistake during Push-Ups is allowing the hips to sag. Your glutes and abs should be tight and your body should be in a relatively straight line throughout the entire movement. Don't allow your hips to sag and touch the ground or raise up to create an arch. If you're having trouble with this, try squeezing your glutes during the movement.

Training Tip

Grip the floor with your fingertips and screw your hands into the ground to create more upper body tension. The added tension will increase shoulder stability, which will help to prevent injuries as well as improve performance.

Easy Does It

Easier: If you struggle with completing a normal Push-Up, give Hand Elevated Push-Ups a try. These are simply Push-Ups with your upper body elevated by placing your hands on a bench or chair. As the Push-Ups become easier, progressively lower the hand elevation until you can start from the floor.

Harder: If regular bodyweight Push-Ups become too easy, you can do Clapping Push-Ups. The Clapping Push-Up is a great exercise to build explosive strength and power. In this exercise, everything stays the same except when you push upward, do so with enough force to lift your hands off the ground. While your hands are off the ground, clap them together in mid-air, "catching" yourself in the top position. From there, return to the bottom and repeat for the desired amount of reps.

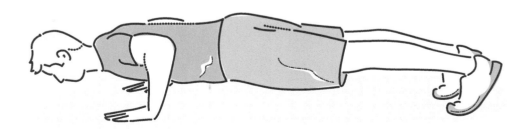

Air Squat

Specific Muscles Involved: Quadriceps, Hamstrings, Glutes

The Air Squat is a fundamental movement. This is always one of the first exercises I teach my clients. This exercise reinforces the squat movement pattern, and is a great workout on its own.

Instructions:

1. Start in a standing position with your feet about shoulder-width apart.

2. Drop your hips down and back like you're sitting in a chair while simultaneously bending your knees. Continue moving down until your hips are below the tops of your knees.

3. Once you reach the bottom position, maintain a vertical torso and stand back up. To help with balance, extend your arms directly out in front of you during the movement.

Easy Does It

Easier: If you struggle reaching depth when squatting, try a Box Air Squat. This is sitting down on a box or bench that requires your knees to reach 90 degrees at the bottom of the movement. Perform Box Air Squats until you feel comfortable without the box or bench for support. Don't relax while sitting on the box; make sure you maintain tension in the core and lower body.

Harder: If you are an Air Squat master, you can replace the Air Squat with the Pistol Squat. The Pistol Squat is an Air Squat on only one leg. These are very challenging and require a great deal of strength and mobility, but they are an excellent goal to aspire to.

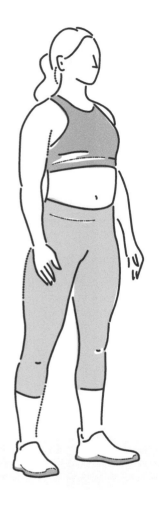

Practice Makes Perfect

The biggest mistake people make is bending forward at the waist during the movement. The goal is to keep the torso as vertical as possible.

Training Tip

Push your knees out during the movement to make sure they stay directly over your toes.

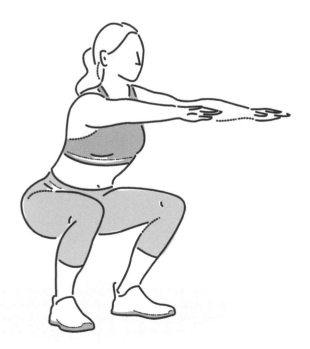

Pull-Up

Specific Muscles Involved: Back

If I had to pick only one back exercise to do for the rest of my life, I would pick the Pull-Up. The Pull-Up is one of the most effective lat-building exercises you can do, and the best part is, all you need is a bar to hang from! These can be done with just your bodyweight, with added weight, or with assistance, depending on your strength level.

Instructions

1. Hang from a fixed overhead bar with a wide overhand grip (palms facing away from your body).

2. Pull yourself up so your chin goes over the bar.

3. Slowly return back to the starting position. Your arms should be straight before beginning another rep.

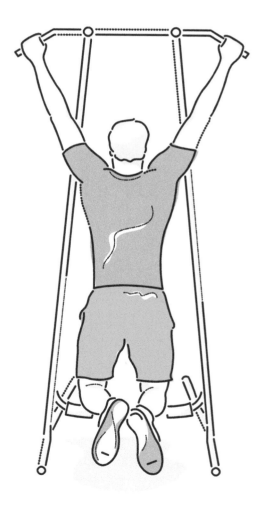

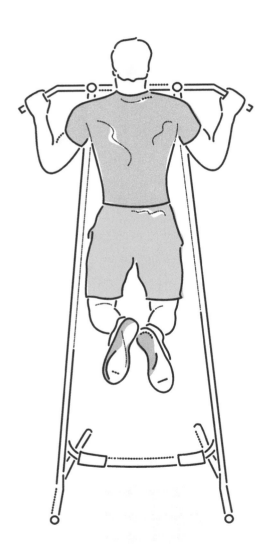

Practice Makes Perfect

With Pull-Ups, the biggest mistake people make is cutting the rep short. This can happen both at the bottom and the top of the movement. Make sure you pull yourself all the way up so that your chin gets above the bar. At the bottom, each rep needs to start with your arms fully straight.

Training Tip

The Pull-Up is very versatile. I recommend using multiple grips—wide, close, neutral, and underhand. If you want to shift a little more emphasis on the biceps, use an underhand grip.

Easy Does It

Easier: The only downside to Pull-Ups is the difficulty. If you struggle with bodyweight Pull-Ups, start with Assisted Pull-Ups by attaching a band to the Pull-Up bar and looping it around your knees. Or, if you have access to one, you can use an Assisted Pull-Up machine.

Harder: Try Weighted Pull-Ups. You can add extra weight via a belt to increase this exercise's intensity.

Flexed Arm Hang

Specific Muscles Involved: Back, Biceps

The Flexed Arm Hang is a movement that has nearly been forgotten in gyms across the United States. What's interesting is that when I was in high school, this was considered a main physical fitness test. I want to do my part in bringing this exercise back! There are a couple of specific benefits. One: The supinated, or underhand, grip (palms facing you) activates biceps more than a traditional pronated, or overhand (palms facing away) Pull-Up grip. This is important because the biceps are hard to train with bodyweight-only exercises. Two: The Flexed Arm Hang is one of the best ways to improve Pull-Up performance.

Instructions

1. Hang from a fixed overhead bar with a narrow underhand grip (palms facing toward your body).

2. Pull yourself (or jump up) into position so your chin goes over the bar. The arms should be flexed, your chest close to the bar, and your legs hanging down straight.

3. Once your chin is over the bar, maintain this position for the duration of the exercise.

Practice Makes Perfect

A common mistake with the Flexed Arm Hang is holding yourself away from the bar. This can actually make the exercise more difficult. Make sure your arms are in a fully flexed position and your chest is held close to the bar.

Training Tip

This exercise can be a little more mentally demanding than most. It's difficult, so you may want to give up early. Focus on your breathing and push through. Listening to music while doing these can help time go by faster.

Easy Does It

Easier: You can do an Assisted Flexed Arm Hang using the band from the Assisted Pull-Ups, or you can place a chair underneath you and use your feet to support some of your bodyweight.

Harder: You can simply hold your Flexed Arm Hangs for longer periods of time.

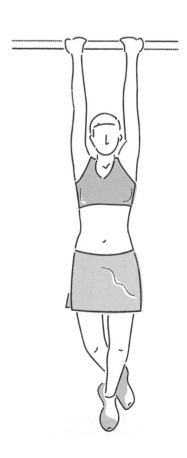
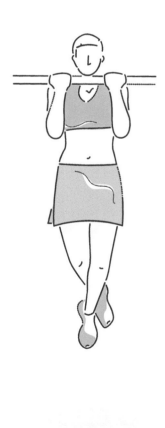

Handstand Push-Up

Specific Muscles Involved: Shoulders

The Handstand Push-Up is one of my all-time favorite exercises for the shoulders. They are just as (if not more effective than) any shoulder exercise done with a dumbbell or barbell. However, they're one of the more difficult bodyweight exercises in this book. Don't let that intimidate you! Unless you have a shoulder injury preventing you from getting into the overhead position, you can do Handstand Push-Ups. Start with the Pike Push-Up (see page 65) if you have to and work from there!

Instructions

1. Face a wall in a standing position. Place your hands about 6 to 12 inches away from the wall on the floor, slightly wider than shoulder-width apart. Make sure your palms are facing away from the wall.

2. Kick your feet up so you're in an overhead handstand position with the wall supporting your feet. Only your heels should be touching the wall.

3. Brace your abs like you are preparing for a punch. Bracing your abs will help maintain a vertical torso.

4. Lower yourself toward the ground until the top of your head lightly touches the floor. Tilting your head back slightly to look toward the ground can help with stability and balance.

5. Once your forehead touches the floor, press yourself up until your elbows reach full extension. Repeat for the desired amount of reps.

Practice Makes Perfect

A common mistake with Handstand Push-Ups is lowering yourself too fast and touching your head on the ground too hard. Be very careful at the bottom of this movement. Hitting your head on the ground too hard can not only hurt the top of your head, but also can be harmful for the spine. Touch the ground with your head as lightly as possible. The extra level of control makes it a more effective exercise as well.

Training Tip

For extra work on the Handstand Push-Up, hold yourself in the top position for **10 seconds** on the last rep. Spending extra time at the top of the Handstand Push-Up helps improve shoulder stability, which ultimately makes you perform the exercise better.

Easy Does It

Easier: **Try a Pike Push-Up. Get into a traditional Push-Up position on the floor. Once in position, raise your hips up, walking your feet toward your hands so that the torso forms an upside-down V. With the top of your head pointing toward the ground, bend your elbows and lower your upper body until the top of your head lightly touches the floor.**

Harder: **None. The Handstand Push-Up is as difficult of a movement as we need to do. If you get to the point where it gets "easy," feel free to add additional reps.**

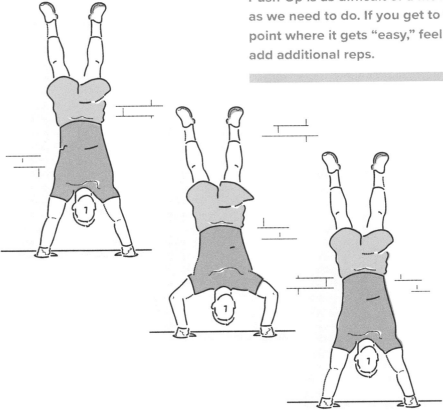

Hanging Leg Raise

Specific Muscles Involved: Abdominals

The problem with many traditional abdominal exercises is they're too easy. This leads to people doing a tremendous amount of reps to "feel the burn." Don't get me wrong; there's nothing bad about knocking out a bunch of reps, but in order to build strength, we need an exercise with increased difficulty. That exercise is the Hanging Leg Raise!

Instructions

1. Grasp an overhead Pull-Up bar with your hands roughly shoulder-width apart, using an overhand (palms facing away) grip.

2. Engage your abdominals and hip flexors to raise your legs outward in front of you, keeping them straight until they're at 90 degrees with your torso, parallel to the ground.

3. Slowly lower your legs to return to the starting position.

Practice Makes Perfect

A common error is allowing too much hip movement during the rep, causing a swinging motion. While performing the movement, aim to keep the torso as still as possible.

Training Tip

Come to a complete stop at the bottom before starting the next rep.

Easy Does It

Easier: Try a Hanging Knee Raise. Instead of raising your full legs up, you can just raise your knees up instead. At the top of the rep, your hips and legs should look like you are sitting in a chair.

Harder: If the Hanging Leg Raise becomes too easy, you can try the full Toes to Bar exercise. With the toes to the bar, instead of stopping once your legs reach 90 degrees, or parallel to the ground, bring them all the way up so your toes come in contact with the bar.

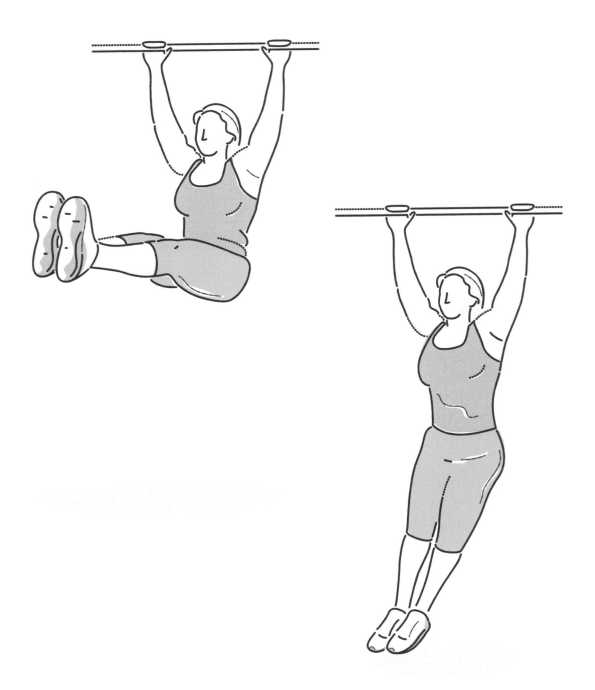

Inverted Row

Specific Muscles Involved: Back

Inverted Rows are one of the most underrated exercises to build upper-back strength. They offer a unique alternative to traditional Machine, Cable, Barbell, and Dumbbell Rows. Also, if you have lower back pain, the Inverted Row is a great way to perform a rowing movement while taking most of the pressure off the low back.

Instructions

1. Position a bar or something to grab onto at about waist height. A kitchen table or desk can work for this.

2. Lie down faceup, with a slightly wider than shoulder-width grip, and position yourself hanging underneath faceup. Your upper and lower body should form a straight line, with your heels on the ground and your arms fully extended.

3. Begin by using your arms and back to pull your chest toward the bar or table. Squeeze your shoulder blades together as you perform the movement. Once your chest comes all the way up to your hands, pause for a second and return yourself back to the starting position.

4. Repeat for the desired number of reps.

Practice Makes Perfect

A common issue people have is keeping their body straight during the movement without letting the hips sag. This requires maintaining tension in the core and glutes.

Training Tip

This is an exercise that gets harder the closer your chest gets to the bar. Make sure you use a full range of motion, going all the way up and all the way down on each rep.

Easy Does It

Easier: The great thing about the Inverted Row is that you can adjust the difficulty simply by raising the bar. The higher the bar, the easier the movement becomes. Just don't raise the bar too high or your feet won't be able to touch the ground!

Harder: If you are looking for more resistance, you can try elevating your feet on a bench to make the movement more difficult.

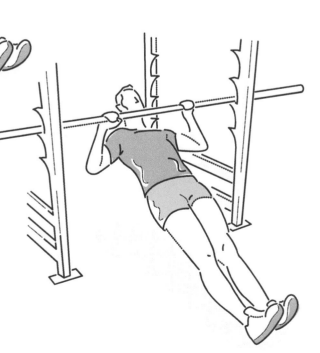

Single-Leg Calf Raise

Specific Muscles Involved: Calves

Not only are strong calves crucial for athleticism, but also they're highly functional. Anyone who has walked up a big hill or carried a heavy box up a few flights of stairs will agree. The best part of the Single-Leg Calf Raise is that it's highly effective and can be done literally anywhere!

Instructions

1. Start off by grasping hold of something or simply placing your palms against a wall for support.

2. Lift one leg off the floor, causing your entire bodyweight to be supported on the other leg.

3. Keep your working leg straight and raise your heel off the ground, lifting your entire bodyweight as you do so.

4. Pause for a second at the top before returning your heel back to the ground. After you complete all the reps on one leg, repeat on the opposite side.

Practice Makes Perfect

The biggest mistake people make with this exercise is going too fast. Take your time and really feel the calf muscles working.

Training Tip

Make sure you use a full range of motion. Try to raise your body up as high as you possibly can on each rep.

Easy Does It

Easier: **Try a Double-Leg Calf Raise.** If using one leg is too difficult at the start, you can use both legs at the same time. The movement pattern is the same; the only difference is that you keep both feet on the ground.

Harder: **Try an Elevated Single-Leg Calf Raise.** If the Single-Leg Calf Raise becomes too easy, a simple way to make the exercise more challenging is to elevate your working foot. This can be done by placing your working foot up on a step. This will allow your heel to get lower, causing a greater range of motion, therefore making the exercise more difficult.

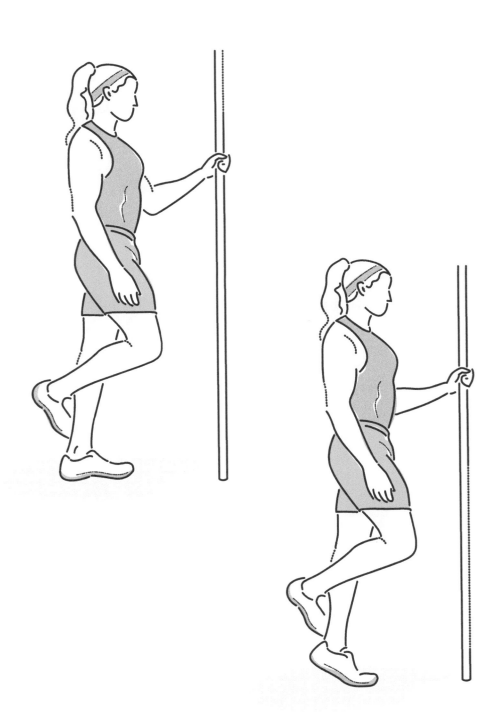

Bench Dips

Specific Muscles Involved: Triceps

The Bench Dip is one of the simplest and most effective triceps exercises you can do. It's also a great transition into eventually doing regular Parallel Bar Dips (see page 80). This is also one of the more versatile exercises in the book, with multiple ways to make it easier or harder.

Instructions

1. For the Bench Dip you will need to stand in front of a bench or chair while facing away from it.

2. Hold on to the bench or chair's edge with arms fully extended and shoulder-width apart. Extend your legs forward, bent at the waist and perpendicular to your torso.

3. Slowly lower your body by bending the elbows. Go down as far as you comfortably can. The greater range of motion you use, the better.

4. Press your torso up, using your triceps, until you reach the starting position.

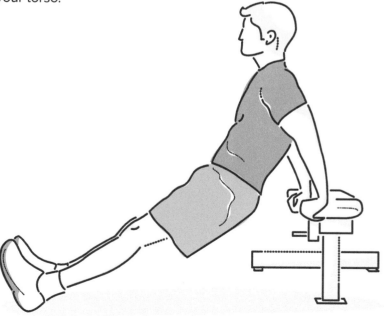

Practice Makes Perfect

Don't allow your hips to shift away from the bench or chair. Try to keep your hips as close as possible by keeping your torso upright.

Training Tip

Keep the elbows tucked as close into your body as possible throughout the movement. This ensures the triceps are the main muscle involved in the movement.

Easy Does It

Easier: Instead of using a bench or chair, you can put your hands on something higher, like a countertop, which will allow you to support less of your bodyweight.

Harder: To make the exercise harder, place your feet up on another bench instead of the ground. Beyond that, you can also place a weight plate on your lap to add extra resistance.

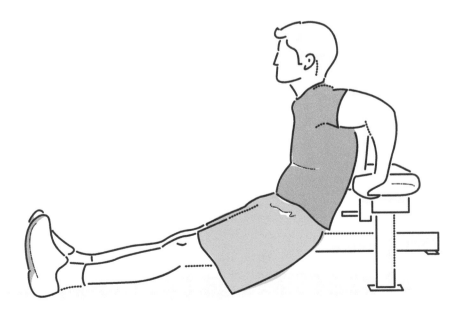

Glute Bridge

Specific Muscles Involved: Glutes

The glutes are the new biceps! It seems like everywhere you look online these days there are glute workouts being marketed left and right, and for good reason. The glutes not only help round out a perfect lower body, but also they're highly functional: Building strong glutes helps you squat and deadlift more weight.

Instructions

1. Begin by lying with your back flat on the floor and your arms down at your sides.

2. To start the movement, drive your hips up toward the ceiling by squeezing your glutes and driving your heels into the floor.

3. Once your hips get as high as possible, hold for a full second before lowering them back to the starting position. Repeat for the desired number of reps.

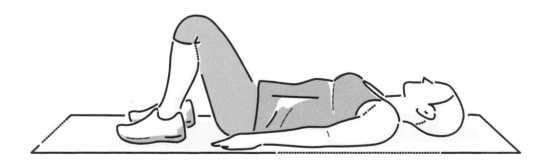

Practice Makes Perfect

The real key with this exercise is trying to get your hips as high as possible. The glutes are activated the most in the end range, so cutting the rep short limits its effectiveness.

Training Tip

Pause and flex your glutes hard at the top of the range of motion.

Easy Does It

Easier: To make the exercise easier, move your feet forward away from your body to cut down the range of motion.

Harder: If the Glute Bridge becomes too easy you can jump up to the Single-Leg Glute Bridge variation. The exercise is done the same way, except you only use one leg at a time.

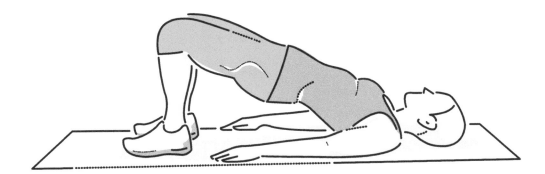

Y-W-T Isohold

Specific Muscles Involved: Shoulders, Back

I love this exercise because it improves your posture. So many of us spend way too much time sitting at our desks or hunched over looking at our phones. This causes our shoulders to round forward and be in that hunched-over position all the time. The Y-W-T Isohold strengthens the posture muscles to help reverse the time spent at our desks and scrolling Instagram.

Instructions

1. Assume a prone (facedown) position on the floor or on a weight bench.

2. By flexing your shoulders and back muscles, hold your arms overhead in a "Y" position, not touching the floor or the weight bench. Hold this position for the desired length of time.

3. Next, lower your hands to create a "W" with your arms and head. Hold this position for the desired length of time.

4. Lastly, move your hands laterally out to your sides to create a "T" position. Hold this position for the desired length of time.

Practice Makes Perfect

Don't allow your hands or arms to touch the floor or bench during the entire exercise. During the movement, aim to raise your arms as high as you can.

Training Tip

Try to build as much tension as possible by flexing your shoulders and back during the exercise.

Easy Does It

Easier: To make the exercise easier, you can cut out one of the positions. Instead of doing a Y-W-T Isohold, you can do a Y-W or a W-T Isohold.

Harder: Hold light objects in each hand, such as soup cans, books, or weight plates.

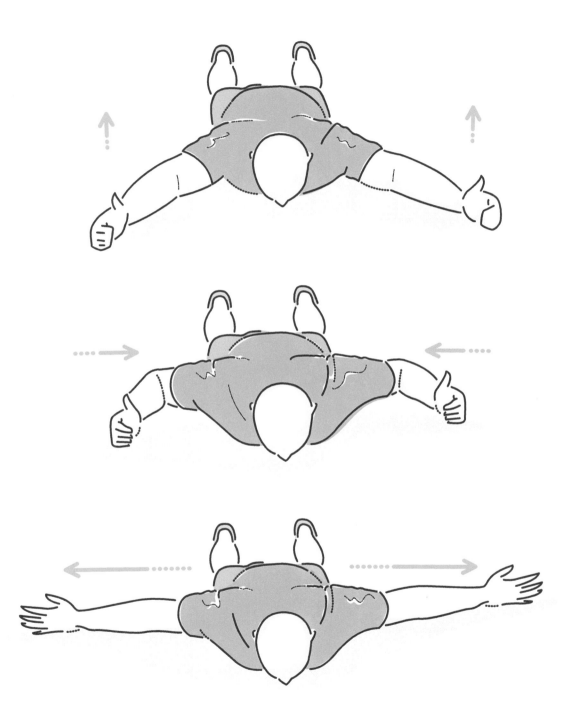

Superman

Specific Muscles Involved: Lower Back

Back pain is very common in today's society. We sit too much and move too little. A weak lower back only makes things worse. The problem most people have is that their lower backs are too weak to perform exercises like the Deadlift (see page 127) safely. Bodyweight exercises are highly underrated for developing muscle and strength. While the lower back is an area of the body that's difficult to properly train without equipment, the Superman is an exception. Using a safe bodyweight exercise like the Superman to improve lower back strength sets you up well to train with weights when your body's ready.

Instructions

1. Begin by lying on the ground facedown, with your arms stretched out above your head, forming a "Y". Keep your legs straight and extended behind you.

2. To start the movement, lift both your arms and legs off the ground at the same time, raising them as high as you can. Keep your head down and look at the floor during the rep.

3. At the top position, you should look like Superman flying. Hold for a full second before returning to the starting position. Repeat for the desired number of reps.

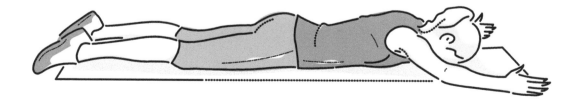

Practice Makes Perfect

Since the Superman has a very short range of motion to begin with, it's important that you aim to raise up as high as you can. Focus specifically on raising your chest and knees, versus your arms and feet.

Training Tip

Keep the head in a neutral position, in line with the spine. If you raise your head up, it could cause you to strain your neck.

Easy Does It

Easier: If the full Superman is too difficult to start with, you can do a Back Extension, which just requires you to lift your chest off the floor while the legs stay down.

Harder: Try the Extended Pause Superman. If the normal Superman exercise becomes too easy, we can add an extended pause at the top of the range of motion. When you lift your legs and arms off the ground, instead of holding the top position for only a full second, hold it for up to 10 seconds each rep. This will add a ton of time under tension, which will increase the difficulty tremendously.

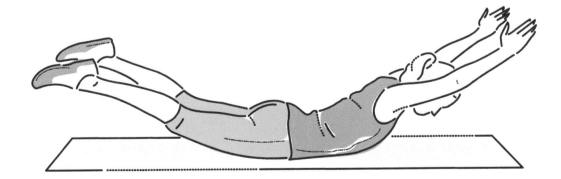

Parallel Bar Dips

Specific Muscles Involved: Chest, Triceps

The Parallel Bar Dip is one of the simplest yet most effective chest and triceps exercises you can do with or without equipment. Most gyms have a set of parallel bars for doing dips. However, if your gym doesn't or if you train at home, you can make do by using the backs of two chairs.

Instructions

1. Stand between a set of parallel bars. Place a hand on each bar, and then take a small jump to help you get into the starting position with your arms locked out.

2. Begin by flexing the elbow and lowering your body until your arms break 90 degrees. To keep the stress on the chest, lean forward about 30 degrees and slightly flare your elbows out to the sides.

3. Reverse the motion by extending the elbow, pushing yourself back up into the starting position.

Practice Makes Perfect

Keep your lower body as still as possible during the exercise. Avoid any leg kicking or swinging to keep all the tension on the upper body.

Training Tip

To put extra emphasis on the chest, use the widest grip you can comfortably perform and lean forward. The closer the grip, and the more vertical the torso stays, the more the triceps engage.

Easy Does It

Easier: If using your bodyweight is too difficult at first, you can use an Assisted Dip Machine. If you don't have an Assisted Dip Machine, Push-Ups are also a great alternative exercise.

Harder: Try Weighted Dips. If you are exceptionally strong on this exercise, you can add a weight belt to create more resistance. Only add weight if moving your bodyweight is too easy. Don't be in a rush to add extra weight before you are ready. For most people, bodyweight dips provide plenty of resistance.

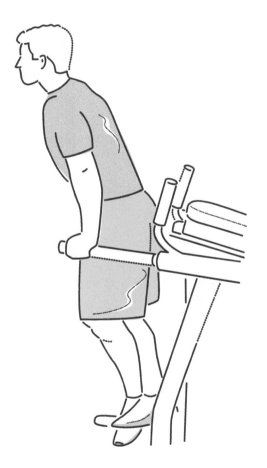

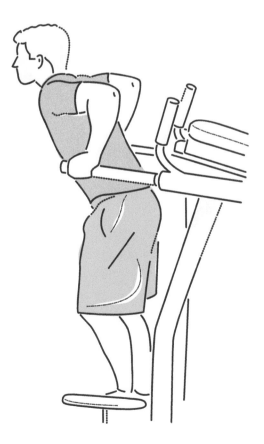

Cossack Squat

Specific Muscles Involved: Quadriceps, Hamstrings, Glutes

The Cossack Squat is a rare bodyweight exercise that most aren't familiar with. It's an advanced bodyweight squat variation that works in the frontal plane (side to side), unlike most lower body exercises. This is a great movement to improve mobility, which can help prevent injuries down the road. Additionally, the Cossack Squat strengthens lower body muscles, like the adductors and hip flexors, that traditional Air Squats do not.

Instructions

1. Start with your feet wider than shoulder-width apart and your toes turned out slightly. How wide your stance will be is determined by your mobility and what feels comfortable. Don't feel like you need to get it dialed in on the first rep. After you do a couple, you may want to move your feet in or out depending on how it feels.

2. Shift your weight toward your right side and begin to sit back, similar to a normal Air Squat. As you are squatting down to the right, lift your left toes off the ground, using your heel as a pivot point. Keep your left leg completely straight.

3. As you squat down, use your arms as a counterbalance by reaching out in front of you. Keep your chest up high throughout the movement.

4. Once you go down as far as you can, stand back up to the starting position.

Practice Makes Perfect

A common mistake with the Cossack Squat is leaning too far forward. Since there is a high mobility demand with this exercise, people often lean forward to help them get down into position. You want to focus on staying as upright as possible.

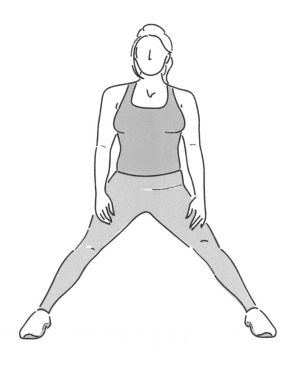

Training Tip

This is one exercise where you can get a great deal of benefit out of it without using a complete range of motion. Only go down as far as you can comfortably and aim to get a little lower each time you do it until you reach below parallel.

Easy Does It

Easier: To make the exercise a little easier to start, you can squat down onto a box or low bench. This is a good way to improve strength and mobility as you work up to being able to do a normal Cossack Squat.

Harder: The only effective way to make the Cossack Squat harder is to add weight. Since the exercise is already pretty challenging, you won't need much. Make sure you hold the weight close to your chest.

Bicycle Crunch

Specific Muscles Involved: Abdominals, Obliques

Bicycle Crunches are very common abdominal exercises, and for good reason. Although the movement is known for being an amazing oblique exercise, Bicycle Crunches actually target your entire core. Speed is the enemy here; make sure you go slow and focus on proper technique.

Instructions

1. Lie on the floor with your lower back pressed into the ground. Place your hands behind your head, with the elbows flared out to the sides. Your knees should be bent at 90 degrees with your feet raised off the floor.

2. Lift your shoulders into the crunch position while simultaneously using a bicycle pedal motion to kick forward with the right leg and retract the left knee. Bring your right elbow close to your left knee by crunching to the side.

3. Go back to the initial starting position.

4. Crunch to the opposite side as you cycle your legs, but this time, lift your left elbow to your right knee.

5. Continue alternating until you've completed all desired reps.

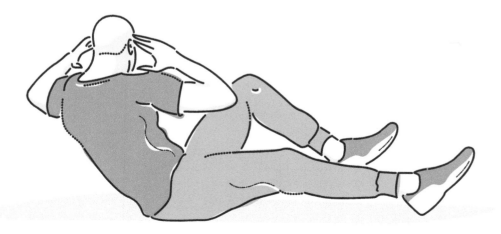

Practice Makes Perfect

A common mistake people make with this movement is rotating their hips on each rep. Your hips should not be rotating; the torso should be doing all of the rotation. Remember to drive your legs straight out while keeping your lower back pressed into the floor for the entire set. Make sure your entire upper body torso is rotating during each rep.

Training Tip

If you feel a strain in your neck while doing this exercise, chances are you are pulling on your neck with your hands. Try doing the exercise with your fingers placed gently behind your ears.

Easy Does It

Easier: If Bicycle Crunches are too difficult, you can start with traditional crunches and go from there!

Harder: Try Side Planks, which are done the same way as regular Planks, except you are on your side and balancing on only one forearm at a time.

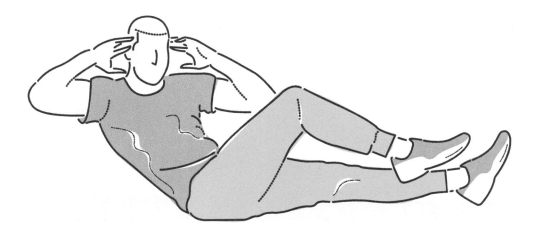

Plank

Specific Muscles Involved: Abdominals

The Plank is an isometric exercise, which means it doesn't require any movement. However, don't let the simplicity of this exercise confuse you. This exercise is very effective. The Plank is a great exercise to improve core stability and prevent lower back pain. Since it doesn't require any actual movement, it's one of the safest core exercises you can do if done correctly.

Instructions

1. Lie facedown on the floor, then lift yourself up using your toes and forearms. Your arms should be bent at 90 degrees with your elbows directly under your shoulders and your wrists aligned with your elbows.

2. Once in position, brace your core hard like you are preparing to take a punch. Flex your glutes and thigh muscles as well while continuing to breathe normally.

3. Keep your body straight at all times and hold this position for the duration of the set.

Practice Makes Perfect

When executing the Plank, it's crucial to keep your body in a straight line at all times. Don't allow your hips to sag or raise due to fatigue. Flex your abs as hard as you can while holding the Plank. This helps maintain good positioning.

Training Tip

Remember to breathe normally during the exercise. It's common to forget to inhale and exhale when creating full-body tension. Additionally, focusing on breathing in regular intervals helps you stay relaxed and keeps your mind off the time remaining.

Easy Does It

Easier: To make the Plank easier, you can do the movement from your knees instead of your toes.

Harder: Try a Feet Elevated One-Leg Plank. To make the Plank more difficult, raise your feet up on a box. To take things to the next level, elevate only one leg at a time. This increases the difficulty.

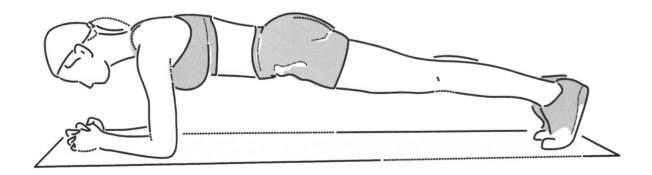

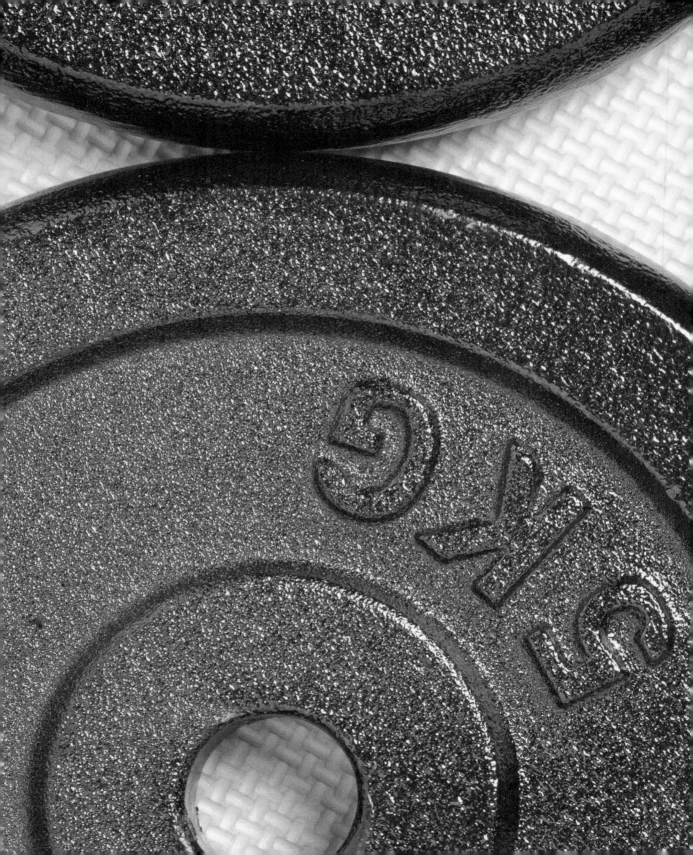

Chapter Six

Dumbbell Exercises

When it comes to strength training, people typically think of barbell training. Barbell training is an excellent way to gain strength, and we'll talk more about barbells later in this book. However, you can absolutely get strong without the stress of the barbell. In fact, dumbbells offer a few unique advantages over barbells. For one, dumbbells are unilateral, which allows each side of the body to work independently. Additionally, dumbbells require greater stabilization, which activates different muscle fibers. It's a lot harder to hide strength imbalances when performing dumbbell exercises. Dumbbell training also results in fewer injuries due to the greater degree of movement freedom and the easier ability to bail if something goes wrong.

Goblet Squat

Specific Muscles Involved: Quadriceps, Hamstrings, Glutes

The Goblet Squat is the perfect introduction to a loaded-squat movement pattern. The Goblet Squat teaches you how to maintain an upright position while dropping into a squat.

Instructions

1. Stand with your feet about shoulder-width apart, holding a dumbbell vertically against your chest (your hands should just be holding the top part of the dumbbell).

2. Drop your hips down and back like you're sitting in a chair while simultaneously bending your knees. Continue until your hips are below the tops of your knees.

3. Once you reach the bottom position, maintain a vertical torso while standing back up to return to your starting position. Your upper body should hardly move during the exercise if you're using your legs, hips, and lower back as one.

Practice Makes Perfect

What you want to remember when performing the Goblet Squat is to make sure the dumbbell is held tight against your chest. This helps reinforce the upright position we want to keep throughout the entire movement.

Training Tip

When dropping into the squat, push your knees out to the sides while keeping your entire foot on the ground. This helps prevent your knees from caving in during the rep.

Easy Does It

Box Goblet Squat: If you struggle reaching depth with the Goblet Squat, try sitting down on a box or bench that requires your knees to reach 90 degrees at the bottom until you feel comfortable without it.

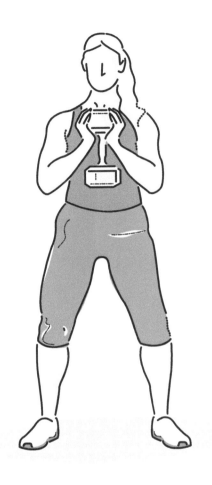

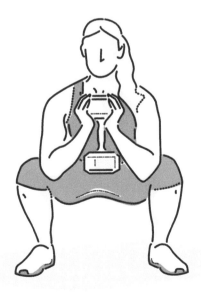

Romanian Deadlift with Dumbbells

Specific Muscles Involved: Hamstrings, Lower Back

The Romanian Deadlift is the best dumbbell exercise to train the posterior chain. It works the same movement pattern as the barbell version, so it's a great alternative when barbells are not accessible. You'll be able to handle quite a bit of weight with these, so make sure you pay attention to proper form to avoid potentially getting hurt.

Instructions

1. Start by holding a pair of dumbbells in front of your hips with your palms facing in toward the body. Your feet should be roughly shoulder-width apart.

2. To begin the movement, push your hips back and lean forward to lower the dumbbells toward your shins. As you are performing this movement, maintain a neutral spine and a slight knee bend. Keep the dumbbells as close to the body as possible.

3. Lower the dumbbells until you reach around mid-shin. You should feel a good stretch in your hamstrings.

4. At the bottom of the range of motion, extend your hips and knees to return back to the starting position.

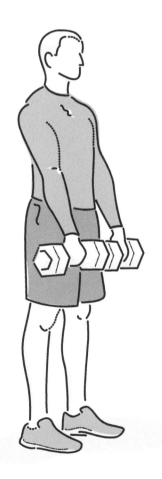

Practice Makes Perfect

A common error with this exercise is rounding the lower back. Let your mobility dictate the range of motion. Only bring the dumbbells down as far as you can while maintaining a neutral spine. Once you start to feel your back round, stop the range of motion there.

Training Tip

Return your dumbbells to the rack in between sets instead of just laying them on the ground. Since you can use heavy dumbbells with this exercise, picking them up from the rack will save your lower back the extra stress.

Easy Does It

Sumo Deadlift: **An easier variation for the dumbbell Romanian Deadlift is a dumbbell Sumo Deadlift. To do this exercise, take a wide stance with toes pointed slightly out and place a dumbbell between your feet. Without rounding your back, drop down and grab one end of a dumbbell with both hands. Once holding the dumbbell, keep knees pushed out and lift it up by straightening your legs and standing up straight.**

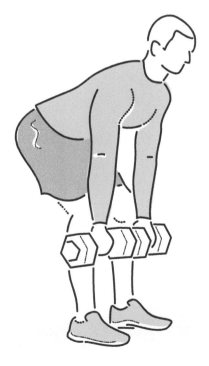

Single-Leg Calf Raise with Dumbbells

Specific Muscles Involved: Calves

When most people think of training calves, they immediately think about using machines, specifically for the standing and seated Calf Raise. However, neither of those exercises are markedly better than a simple Single-Leg Calf Raise with Dumbbells. If done correctly, this movement is extremely effective.

Instructions

1. Start off by grasping hold of something for support, and then, with the nonsupporting hand, hold a dumbbell.

2. Lift one leg off the floor. Your entire bodyweight should be supported by the other leg. Be sure that the dumbbell and the leg supporting your bodyweight are on the same side of the body.

3. Keep your working leg (the one supporting your bodyweight) straight and raise your heel off the ground, lifting your bodyweight as you do so.

4. Pause for a second at the top before returning your heel back to the ground. After you complete all the reps on one leg, repeat on the opposite side.

Practice Makes Perfect

A common mistake is using too much weight. This causes you to be unable to get a full extension at the top. Only use a weight with which you can move through a full range of motion.

Training Tip

Flex your calf when you pause at the top of the range of motion.

Easy Does It

Standing Calf Raise with Dumbbells: If the single-leg variation is too difficult, you can keep both feet on the ground and use both legs at the same time. The movement pattern is the same.

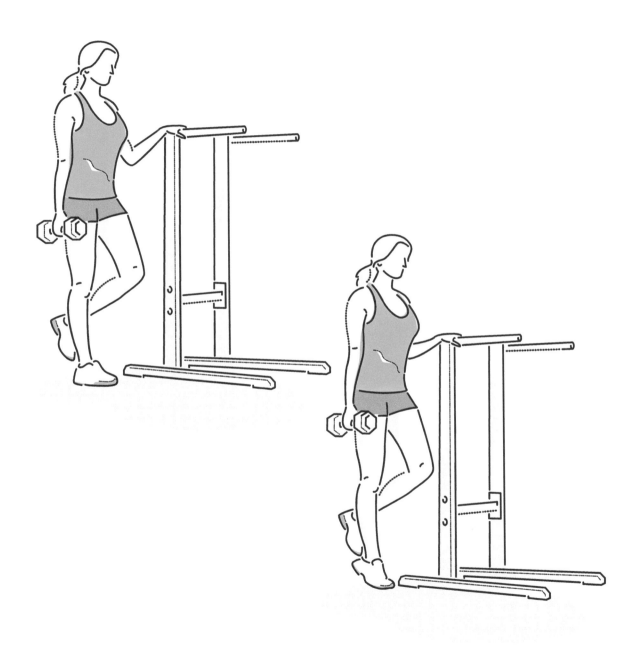

Weighted Lunges

Specific Muscles Involved: Quadriceps, Hamstrings, Glutes

The Weighted Lunge is one of the most popular lower body exercises and one of my all-time favorites. One of the biggest benefits to this movement is that it works on balance as well as muscular strength. Getting strong through Weighted Lunges is a true testament of functional strength.

Instructions

1. Stand holding two dumbbells, one in each of your hands by your sides.

2. Step forward two feet with the right leg and lower your upper body. The torso should stay upright. Maintain your balance.

3. Push into the heel of your forward foot to return to the starting position.

4. Repeat for the desired amount of reps, then switch sides and perform with the opposite leg.

Practice Makes Perfect

If you take too big of a step, it becomes hard to maintain balance. Both legs should be bent roughly 90 degrees in the bottom position of the movement.

Training Tip

Use a full range of motion. Make sure you are touching your back knee to the ground during each rep.

Easy Does It

Bodyweight Lunges: If Weighted Lunges are too difficult at first, feel free to use just your bodyweight.

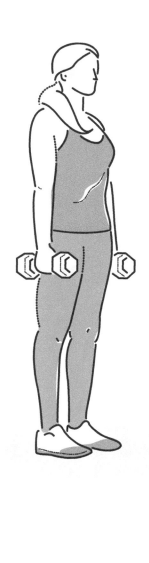
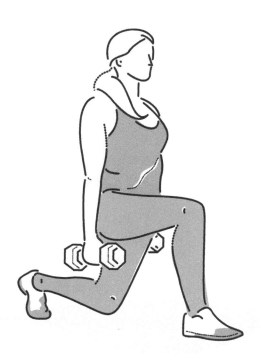

Flat Bench Press with Dumbbells

Specific Muscles Involved: Chest

This dumbbell Bench Press variation allows for both sides of the chest to be worked equally, which can reveal any imbalance issues you may have. Dumbbells also allow for a greater range of motion than a barbell. I also like the fact that you can go heavy with these without needing a spotter!

Instructions

1. Sit on the edge of a bench with a dumbbell in each hand, with the dumbbells resting on top of your knees. The palms of your hands should be facing each other.

2. Keep the dumbbells close to your chest and roll back onto the bench so you are lying down on it, faceup. From there, position the dumbbells out to your sides, next to your shoulders.

3. Once you have the dumbbells in position, make sure the palms of your hands are facing away from you. This is the starting position.

4. To begin the movement, push the dumbbells up until both arms are straight.

5. Once you reach the end range of motion, with both arms fully extended, slowly lower the weight back to the starting position and repeat for the desired amount of reps.

Practice Makes Perfect

One of the benefits of using dumbbells is the greater range of motion these weights allow. However, because there is not a definitive end point like there is with a barbell Bench Press (bar touching chest), it's easy to cut the rep short. Make sure you're always using a full range of motion (unless an injury causes you to do otherwise).

Training Tip

You can start each rep from the top or bottom depending on what's most comfortable for you.

Easy Does It

Push-Ups: If you don't have access to dumbbells light enough to perform the Flat Bench Press, an easy alternative is to just replace them with Push-Ups (see page 56).

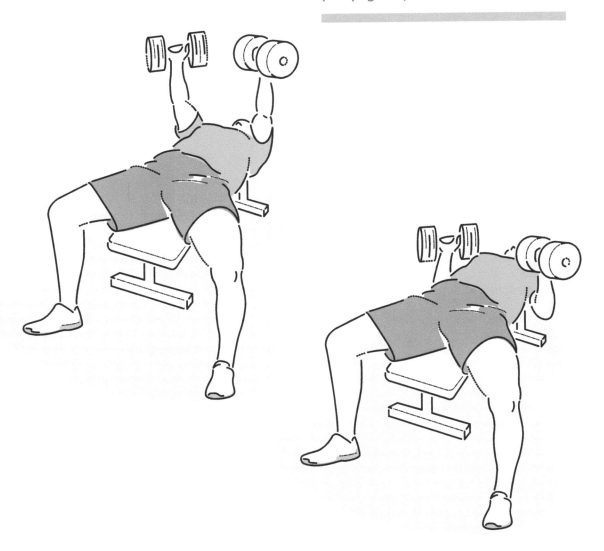

Incline Bench Press with Dumbbells

Specific Muscles Involved: Chest

The Incline Bench Press is very similar to the Flat Bench Press (see page 98), but the inclined bench angle shifts the focus to the upper chest, near your collarbone. Similar to the flat variation, the Incline Bench Press also allows for both sides of the chest to be worked equally, which can prevent imbalance issues. This is my favorite incline variation to work the upper part of the chest because the barbell variety tends to be hard on the shoulders for some people. Adjust the bench angle to find what works best for you. Use an angle less than 45 degrees if possible.

Instructions

1. Sit on the edge of a bench with a dumbbell in each hand. The dumbbells should be resting on top of your knees, and the palms of your hands should be facing each other.

2. To get the dumbbells into position, use your knees to help kick the dumbbells up to your shoulders. To make it easier, kick each dumbbell up one at a time.

3. Once you have both dumbbells at shoulder level, rotate your wrists forward so palms are facing away from you.

4. Push the dumbbells up until both arms are straight.

5. Once you reach the end range of motion, with both arms fully extended, slowly lower the weights back to the starting position and repeat for the desired amount of reps.

Practice Makes Perfect

If you arch your back too much, it takes the tension off the upper chest and defeats the purpose of the exercise. It's okay to have your shoulders retracted, but try to limit excessive arching.

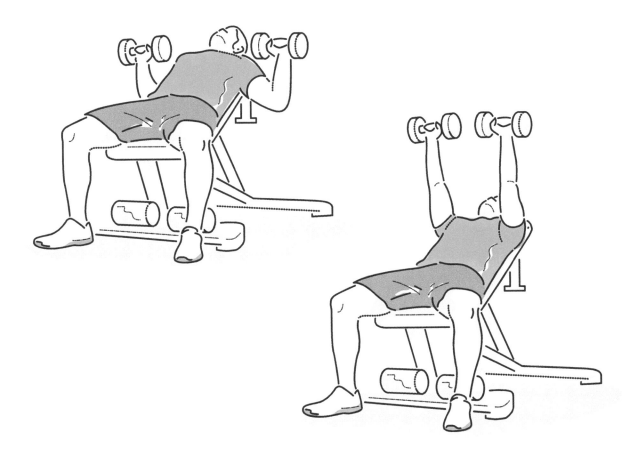

Training Tip

If you have a gym partner, have them help you get the dumbbells into position. Also, if it feels more comfortable, you can press the dumbbells straight up with a neutral grip (palms facing each other) instead of using a pronated grip.

Easy Does It

Incline Hammer Strength Machine Press: Using an Incline Hammer Strength Machine Press is an easier variation to work the upper chest region since you don't have to worry about stabilizing the dumbbells. With this exercise, all you have to do is adjust the seat and weight, sit down, and press.

Weighted Sit-Up

Specific Muscles Involved: Abdominals

Sit-Ups are fundamental abdominal exercises to help build a strong core. But there comes a point where they become too easy. Instead of just adding an endless amount of reps, the better option is to add weight.

Instructions

1. Start by lying down on your back with your knees bent 90 degrees and feet flat on the floor.

2. Grab a dumbbell with both hands and hold it tight up against your chest.

3. Engage the core and raise your upper torso until the backs of your forearms touch your legs. Slowly lower yourself to the ground, maintaining control.

Practice Makes Perfect

A common mistake people make is allowing their feet to come off the floor. It helps if you have something or someone to help anchor them to the ground.

Training Tip

Hold the dumbbell up against your chest, not out in front of you.

Easy Does It

Regular Sit-Up: If the dumbbell Weighted Sit-Up is too difficult to start with, you can simply perform a regular Sit-Up until you build up the strength to be able to add weight.

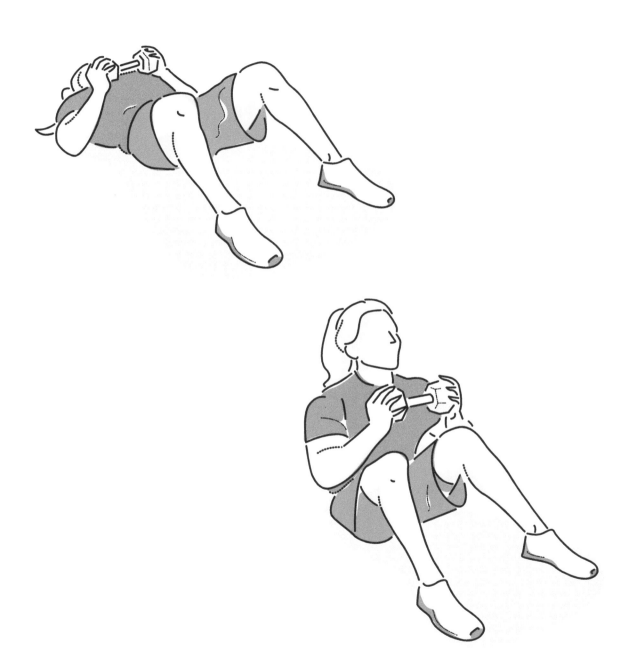

Side Bend

Specific Muscles Involved: Abdominals, Obliques

There was a time when this exercise fell out of favor with the fitness community due to some misinformation. It was thought that doing Side Bends, which work the sides of your midsection (obliques), would make your waist larger. The truth is, no one ever complained about having lean and muscular love handles. An excess layer of body fat causes unwanted waist expansion, not building muscular obliques.

Instructions

1. Hold a dumbbell in one hand while standing with your feet shoulder-width apart. Brace your core.

2. Bend at the waist toward the side of your body holding the dumbbell. Lower the dumbbell as far as you can, keeping your abs braced the entire time.

3. Hold the bottom position for a moment before returning to the starting position.

4. Repeat on the opposite side.

Practice Makes Perfect

Do not lean forward during the movement. All of the movement should be side to side.

Training Tip

Don't hold dumbbells in both hands thinking you can save time by doing the reps back-to-back. This actually makes the exercise easier as the second dumbbell counterbalances the working side.

Easy Does It

Unweighted Side Bends: If holding a light dumbbell is too challenging at first, you can do these without weights until you get the hang of the movement pattern. Follow the movement steps listed here without the dumbbell.

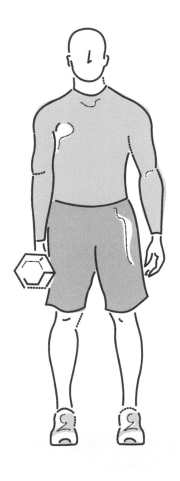

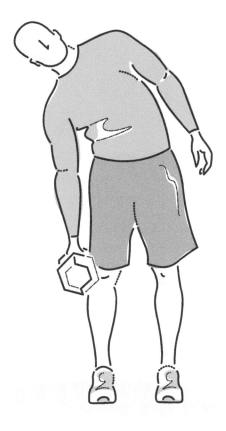

Standing Shoulder Press

Specific Muscles Involved: Shoulders

The Standing Shoulder Press is right up there with the Handstand Push-Up (see page 64) and Overhead Press (see page 142) as one of the best overall shoulder strength builders. The dumbbell version allows your hands to move freely since they're not fixed to a barbell. This helps prevent shoulder injuries. Using dumbbells also allows you to work each side individually, which helps eliminate muscular imbalances.

Instructions

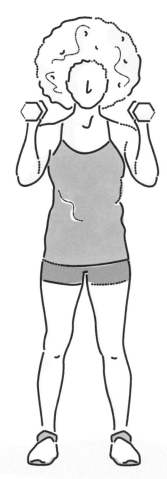

1. Start by holding a dumbbell in each hand at shoulder height with your palms facing forward.

2. Stand straight, feet shoulder-width apart, with your abs braced and with a slight bend in the knees.

3. While keeping your back straight, press the weights up above the head in a controlled motion.

4. Once the arms are fully extended, slowly return the dumbbells back down to the starting position.

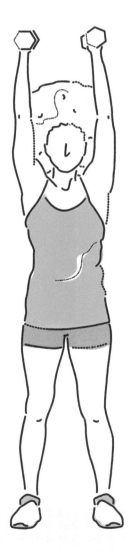

Practice Makes Perfect

A common mistake people make with the Standing Shoulder Press is leaning back and allowing the lower back to arch. Remain standing straight up with the core braced during the entire movement.

Training Tip

Keep the wrists as straight as possible while pressing the dumbbells. If the wrists bend back, it can limit how much weight you can use.

Easy Does It

Seated Shoulder Press: The seated version is a great alternative if you have lower back pain. Use an adjustable bench that allows you to sit up straight and press the dumbbells over your head.

Side Raise

Specific Muscles Involved: Shoulders

This may surprise you, but the dumbbell Side Raise is one of the most irreplaceable exercises in this book. No other exercise trains the side of the shoulder the way the Side Raise does. If you see someone with impressive shoulders, chances are they have spent a lot of time doing dumbbell Side Raises. From a functional standpoint, have you ever carried the garbage out and struggled to lift the bag up and over into the garbage can? Dumbbell Side Raises will help make that much easier!

Instructions

1. Stand with a straight back, rib cage down, holding one dumbbell in each hand. To bring your rib cage down, brace your core like you're getting ready for a punch. This is the starting position.

2. Leading with the elbows slightly bent, raise the dumbbells to the side until your arms are parallel to the ground.

3. Pause for one second before returning to the starting position.

Practice Makes Perfect

A common mistake people make is shrugging their shoulders on the upward part of the movement. This takes some of the tension off of the side delt and puts it into the traps. Keep the shoulders retracted and locked down. The goal is to keep all of the movement in the arms.

Training Tip

To maintain the correct arm positioning, lead with your elbows versus with your hands.

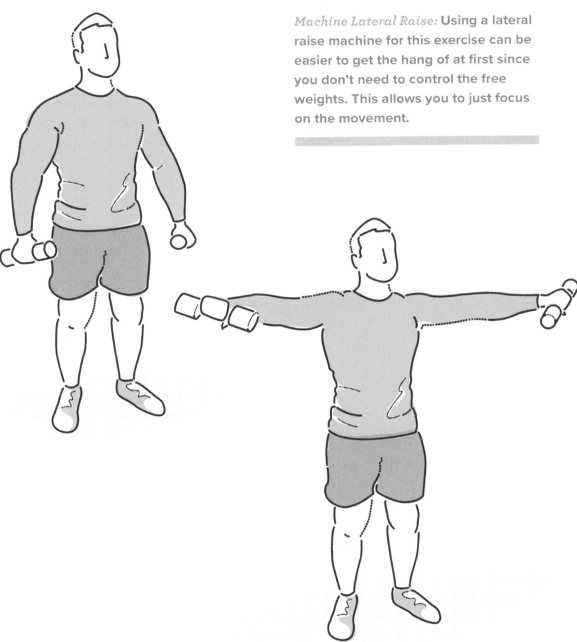

Easy Does It

Machine Lateral Raise: Using a lateral raise machine for this exercise can be easier to get the hang of at first since you don't need to control the free weights. This allows you to just focus on the movement.

Hammer Curl

Specific Muscles Involved: Biceps, Forearms

The dumbbell Hammer Curl is one of the best all-around biceps exercises you can do. What's unique about the Hammer Curl is the neutral grip. This incorporates the brachialis, a muscle between the biceps and triceps, and also incorporates some forearm as well. Forearm and grip strength are among the most fundamental strengths that our day-to-day lives require.

Instructions

1. Stand straight, holding one dumbbell in each hand using a closed, neutral grip (palms facing body). Position the dumbbells along your thighs with your arms fully extended. This is the starting position.

2. Maintaining the neutral grip, curl the dumbbells toward your shoulders. Pay attention to your elbows' positions. Your elbows should remain steady at your side throughout the entire rep. Avoid letting them drift forward during the movement.

3. Once executed, lower the weights until your arms are fully extended.

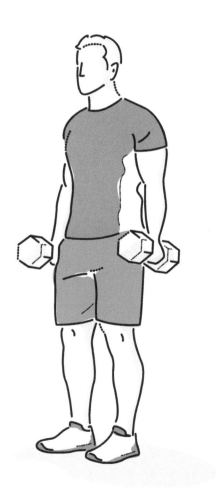

Practice Makes Perfect

If the weight is too heavy, it's common for the elbow to drift forward or out to the sides during the rep. This takes the tension off the biceps and shifts it to the shoulders. You want to lock the elbows in place for the duration of the set.

Training Tip

To focus more on each arm, perform one arm at a time.

Easy Does It

Concentration Curl: If the dumbbell Hammer Curl doesn't work well for you, you can replace it with a dumbbell Concentration Curl. Sit at the edge of a bench with your knees bent and feet flat on the floor. While holding a dumbbell, brace your arm against the inside of your thigh. Your hand should be down by the floor. Perform the movement by curling the dumbbell up toward your shoulder.

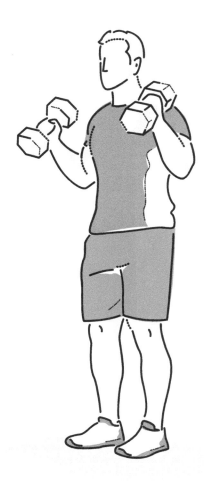

Alternating Curl

Specific Muscles Involved: Biceps

Over the years, I've found the simple exercises are often the ones done incorrectly. The dumbbell Alternating Curl falls into that category. If you hand someone a pair of dumbbells and tell them to start lifting them, most likely they will begin to curl them. The dumbbell Alternating Curl is a fundamental exercise, but the key is making sure we get the most out of it.

Instructions

1. Start by standing in a shoulder-width stance, holding a dumbbell in each hand. Position your hands so that your palms are facing in toward the body.

2. Curl the dumbbell in your right hand up by bending at the elbow and lifting it toward your shoulder. As you curl the weight, rotate your wrist so that your palm is facing up at the top of the rep. Avoid bending at the waist or leaning back when you are curling the weight up.

3. Once you curl the dumbbell as far up as you can, slowly lower it back to the starting position.

4. After you complete the rep on the right side, complete a rep on the left side. Continue alternating back and forth for the desired number of reps.

Practice Makes Perfect

The biggest issue people have when performing the Alternating Curl with dumbbells is allowing their elbow to move forward or out to the side. Keep your elbow locked in place, pointing down toward the floor, and close to the torso during the entire rep.

Training Tip

Squeeze your biceps hard at the top of the rep. This will accentuate the "pump" feeling.

Easy Does It

Dumbbell Curl: Aside from lowering the weight on the Alternating Curl, you can also make the exercise easier by curling both dumbbells up at the same time. Start by holding a dumbbell in each hand with the palms facing up toward the ceiling. To perform the movement, simply curl both dumbbells straight up.

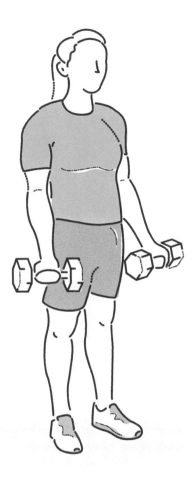

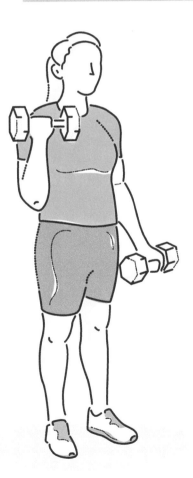

Triceps Kickback

Specific Muscles Involved: Triceps

This is one exercise where you want to make sure you keep your ego in check. The correct weight is often a little less than you would expect. Our goal with the Triceps Kickback is not to move a ton of weight but to build the triceps as best we can.

Instructions

1. Place your left knee on the bench with your left palm flat on the bench. Have a dumbbell on the ground on the right side of the bench.

2. Pick up the dumbbell with your right hand using an overhand grip. Your palm should be facing the bench.

3. Raise your arm until it's in line with the body, keeping your elbow tucked into your side and bent at a 90-degree angle.

4. Keep your upper arm still and extend your forearm until it creates a straight line with your shoulder.

5. Once your arm is in full extension, hold for a second before slowly returning back to the starting position.

6. After completing the desired number of reps, repeat on the opposite side.

Practice Makes Perfect

The most common error with the Triceps Kickback happens with elbow positioning. You want to make sure the elbow is at the same level as the shoulder, and your upper arm is parallel with the ground. If the elbow is higher or lower than the shoulder, this exercise becomes less effective.

Training Tip

Flex your triceps hard at the top of the range of motion and hold the position for a full second. Don't rush to lower the weight.

Easy Does It

Bench Dips: The dumbbell Triceps Kickback can be hard to position correctly at first. If you are struggling, you can do Bench Dips (see page 72) instead.

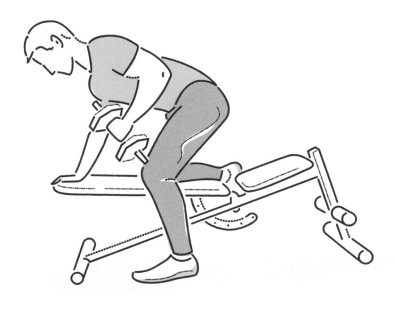

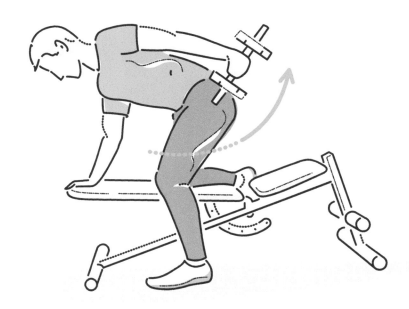

Overhead Triceps Extension with Dumbbells

Specific Muscles Involved: Triceps

The Overhead Triceps Extension with Dumbbells is one of the best triceps builders we can do. Unlike the dumbbell Triceps Kickback (see page 114), this is an exercise in which we can use a lot of weight, making it great at developing strength.

Instructions

1. Stand with your feet shoulder-width apart and your core braced. Hold a dumbbell with both hands behind your head.

2. Extend the dumbbell over your head until your arms are fully extended.

3. Once your arms are fully extended, hold for a second before slowly returning the dumbbell back to the starting position.

Practice Makes Perfect

To keep as much tension on the triceps as possible, you want to prevent the elbows from flaring out too far to the sides. The elbows should be facing forward during the entire rep.

Training Tip

Let the dumbbell travel as low as possible on each rep to get a big stretch in the triceps.

Seated Overhead Triceps Extension with Dumbbells: **This is a variation that can take some pressure off the lower back. If you have lower back pain or experience lower back pain doing this exercise standing, try sitting on the edge of a bench with feet flat on the floor to perform the exercise.**

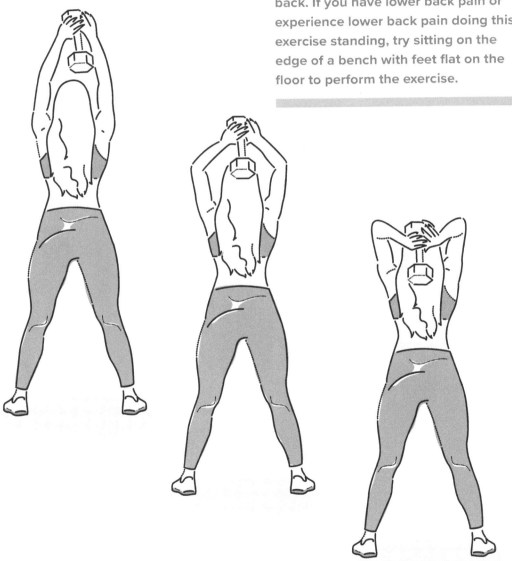

Dumbbell Row

Specific Muscles Involved: Back

I like the Dumbbell Row because it allows us to work on each side individually. Also, because of the unilateral nature of the exercise, we can brace the upper body with one hand while rowing with the other. Being able to brace takes some of the pressure off of the lower back.

Instructions

1. Grab a dumbbell with the palm facing in toward your body. Place the opposite hand and knee on the bench or chair for support.

2. Keeping your back straight, pull the dumbbell up and back toward your hip, trying to get the dumbbell as high as possible.

3. At the top of the movement, allow the shoulder blades to move and retract in order to get the full range of motion.

4. Repeat on the opposite side.

Practice Makes Perfect

People tend to rotate their torso during the movement because it makes them feel like they're going through a greater range of motion. In reality, torso rotation limits lat activation.

Training Tip

It's common for people to use too much weight and end up using every muscle except the back to move the dumbbell. Remember, there is no trophy handed out to the strongest dumbbell rower. Use a weight you can handle. Pause the dumbbell at the top for a second or two to make the exercise harder and to maximize the muscle contraction.

Easy Does It

Chest-Supported Incline Row: This is a great alternative to the Dumbbell Row. Using the support of the incline bench takes some pressure off of the lower back. Start by setting an adjustable bench at a 30- to 45-degree angle. Place two dumbbells on the floor at the bottom of the bench. Lean into the bench, facedown, while grasping a dumbbell in each hand. Begin with the arms hanging down toward the floor and perform the movement by rowing the dumbbells up to your sides.

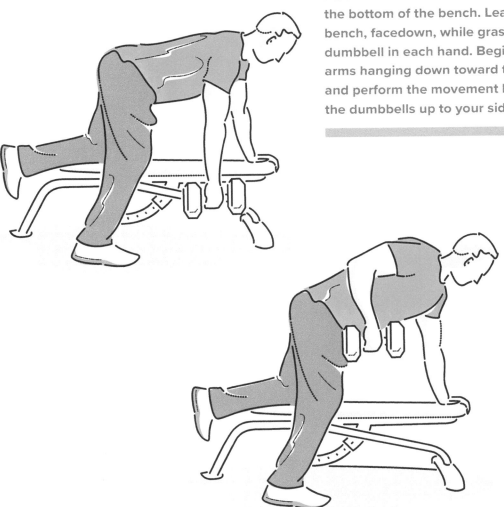

Dumbbell Pullover

Specific Muscles Involved: Chest, Back

Watch any video of Arnold Schwarzenegger training in the 1970s and you'll most likely see him performing Dumbbell Pullovers. I consider the Pullover an "old-school" exercise because you don't see it done much anymore. It's a shame this exercise fell out of favor, because it's a unique chest and back combo exercise that also works the serratus. The Dumbbell Pullover is also one of the few chest exercises that doesn't involve pressing, so it's easier on the elbows.

Instructions

1. Stand a dumbbell up vertically on a flat bench so you can easily grab it.

2. Lie with your legs perpendicular to the bench and keep only your shoulders and upper back on the surface. Your head should be off the bench, and your hips should be below the bench with legs bent.

3. Hold the dumbbell with your palms pressing the underside. Slightly bending your arms, raise it above your chest.

4. While keeping arms locked in the starting position, slowly lower the weight in an arc behind your head until you feel a good stretch across your chest.

5. Bring the dumbbell back in the same curving motion to the starting position.

Practice Makes Perfect

If the arms are bent too much during this movement, it can become more of a triceps exercise, which is not what you are looking for. The key is to maintain the same arm angle throughout the duration of the exercise.

Training Tip

Get a good stretch in the bottom position; really try to "open up" your rib cage. As you pull the dumbbell up, flex the chest hard at the top.

Easy Does It

Machine Pullover: **Some gyms have a pullover machine, but keep in mind that the machine tends to target the lats a little more than the chest. Adjust the seat so that your arms are flat on the pads and you are able to grasp the bar above with both hands while sitting. Pull the bar down, driving your arms and elbows into the pads. Pull down as far as the machine allows, then slowly bring the weight back to the starting position.**

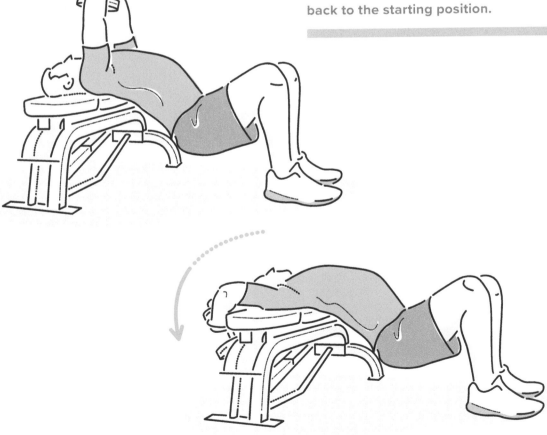

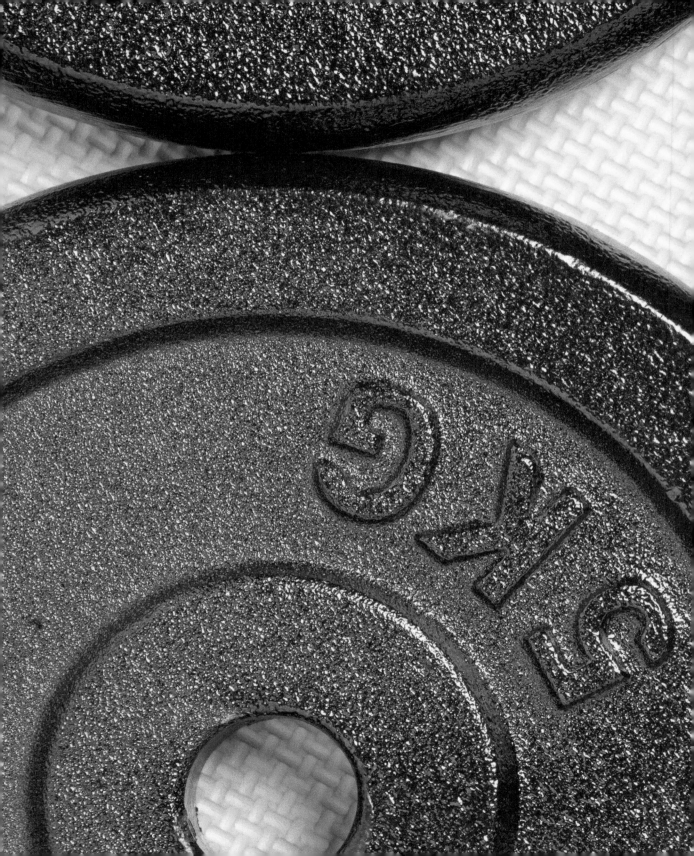

Chapter Seven

Barbell Exercises

Although bodyweight and dumbbell exercises are very effective, the barbell is the undisputed king of strength. Strength is best built using high resistance and a lower amount of rep sets that place the muscles under high levels of tension. This makes barbells perfect for strength building since they offer the ability to handle more weight than any other strength training implement. The results speak for themselves; no other implement is responsible for developing more total body strength in the history of resistance training. The key with barbell training is using proper form to get the most out of the exercises and prevent injuries.

Back Squat

Specific Muscles Involved: Quadriceps, Hamstrings, Glutes

There's a reason the Back Squat is often referred to as the "king of all exercises." The Back Squat uses nearly the entire muscular system, developing the lower body like no other exercise. If I could only pick one movement to have in the program, the Back Squat would be at the top of the list.

Instructions

The Setup

1. Start with the barbell resting in a stand around chest level.

2. Grab the bar with a slightly wider than shoulder-width grip.

3. With a tight grip, step under the bar, and position feet parallel to each other.

4. Squeeze your shoulder blades together to create a shelf where the bar can rest. Place the bar in a balanced position across the upper back and shoulders.

5. Once the bar is set, take a deep breath, brace your core, and extend your hips and knees to lift the bar from the rack.

6. After you remove the barbell from the stand, take two short steps straight back. Your feet should end up in a slightly wider than shoulder-width stance. Most people will benefit from having their toes pointed out to a small degree. This is the starting position.

The Back Squat

7. Take a deep breath, brace your core, and begin the descent.

8. Bend at the knees while dropping your hips back until the tops of your thighs are parallel to the ground.

9. The moment you reach parallel, stand back up to the starting position.

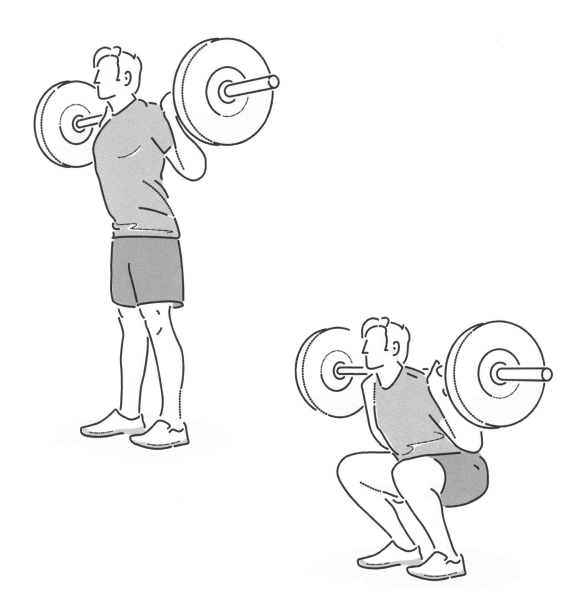

continued

Practice Makes Perfect

Knee cave is one of the most common issues people have while squatting. This is when the knees move toward each other during the upward motion of the squat. Over time, this could potentially lead to knee pain or even a knee injury. There are two things we can do to address this issue:

Change Foot Width: If the starting foot position is too wide, the body will compensate by bringing the knees toward each other. Try bringing your stance in closer to shoulder-width position.

Drive the Knees Out: A common coaching cue to improve knee tracking is simply to focus on driving the knees out during the lift. Sometimes just being mindful of knee position helps take care of the problem.

Training Tip

Unlike most lifting exercises, the type of shoes we wear when squatting is important. Ideally, we want something with a hard, flat surface. Converse Chuck Taylors or most Vans fit the bill. Another option is to use an Olympic weightlifting shoe specifically designed for squatting. These have elevated heels, which can help you maintain an upright posture while squatting at or below parallel.

Most importantly, we want to avoid squatting in running shoes at all costs. The soft sole in most running shoes is like trying to squat on a pillow. This is great for running but not for squatting.

Easy Does It

Goblet Squat: If you are not comfortable using a barbell yet, you can stick with the Goblet Squat (see page 90).

Deadlift

Specific Muscles Involved: Hamstrings, Glutes, Back

The Deadlift is a great exercise to build muscle and strength along the entire posterior chain (back, hamstrings, and glutes). It is also one of the most functional exercises we can do in the gym. The act of picking things up off the ground is something we all do daily.

Instructions

The Setup

1. Stand facing a barbell, with the feet about shoulder-width apart. The shins should be a couple inches away from the bar while standing. Another way to look at it is that the bar should cut the foot in half.

2. Squat down with the hips lower than the shoulders and grab the bar. The hands should be outside of the knees and the elbows should be fully extended. The arms stay locked out throughout the entire movement.

3. At the bottom, the back should be flat or slightly arched, and the hips should be above the knees, creating tension in the hamstrings. This is the starting position.

The Deadlift

4. Take a deep breath, brace your core, and lift the bar from the floor by extending the hips and knees.

5. The torso angle should remain constant; avoid letting the hips rise before the shoulders. The back should remain flat.

6. As the bar is being raised, keep it as close to the body as possible.

7. Once the bar passes the knees, drive the hips forward, extend the legs, and finish with the shoulders behind the bar and the body standing straight up.

8. With a straight back, return the bar to the starting position.

continued

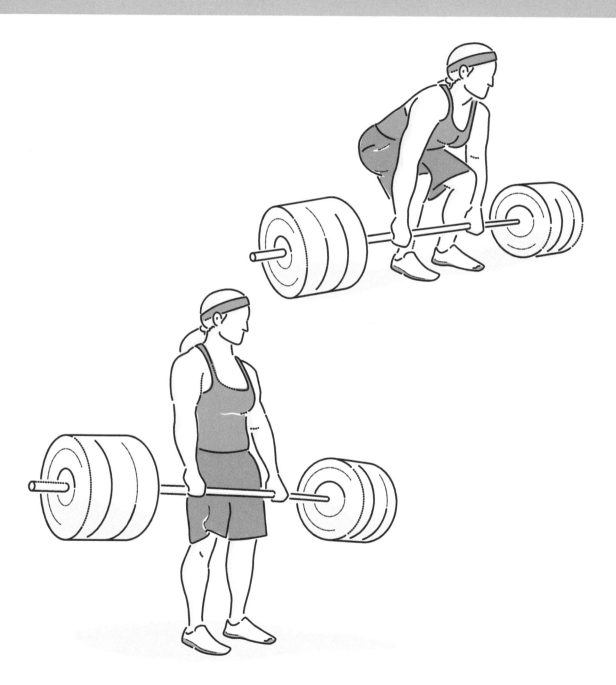

Practice Makes Perfect

The biggest mistake anyone can make while deadlifting is allowing the back to round. This can be caused by multiple factors, but the most common is a lack of tension on the bar before starting the lift. Before even lifting the weight off the ground, it's important to create tension on the bar. Some coaches like to call this "taking the slack out." Once in the starting position, pull the bar up only enough to apply upward pressure, but not enough to lift the weight off the ground. This is maybe 5 to 10 percent of the force necessary to actually lift the weight. What this does is it helps get your muscles activated and ready before lifting the weight. This prevents the hips from shooting up early and causing the back to round.

Training Tip

If you find it hard to hang on to the bar during the lift, you can use what is called a mixed grip to prevent the bar from rolling out of your hands. To use a mixed grip, place one hand over the bar like normal (pronated) and reverse the grip and grab the bar underhand (supinated) with your other hand.

Easy Does It

Trap Bar Deadlift: The traditional barbell Deadlift can be difficult to master when you're first starting out. A great alternative is a Trap Bar Deadlift. The movement pattern is nearly the same, but the handles are at your sides and higher, allowing you to get into a better starting position.

Hip Thrust

Specific Muscles Involved: Glutes

The barbell Hip Thrust is arguably the best glute-building exercise there is. If you want to maximize glute development, including the barbell Hip Thrust is a must. The benefits don't stop with just aesthetics either; glute strength plays a role in many athletic movements.

Instructions

The Setup

1. Place your upper back on a bench with a barbell laying across your hips. Hold the barbell in place with both hands. Keep your feet planted firmly on the ground out in front of you at about shoulder-width. This is the starting position.

The Hip Thrust

2. Drive your hips up toward the sky, engaging your glutes at the top. Perform the movement slowly, exercising control. It's a small range of motion, so make sure you raise your hips as high as you can.

3. Once you reach full extension, hold for a count then lower back to the starting position.

Practice Makes Perfect

Since the barbell Hip Thrust has a limited range of motion to begin with, it's important to extend your hips fully at the top and use the maximum range of motion. The glutes are most activated at the top of the rep, so cutting the range of motion short limits the effectiveness of this exercise.

Training Tip

You can use a thick pad or wrap a towel around the barbell to prevent it from digging into your hips when you thrust.

Easy Does It

Glute Bridge: If the barbell is too difficult to start with, you can stick to the bodyweight Glute Bridge (see page 74).

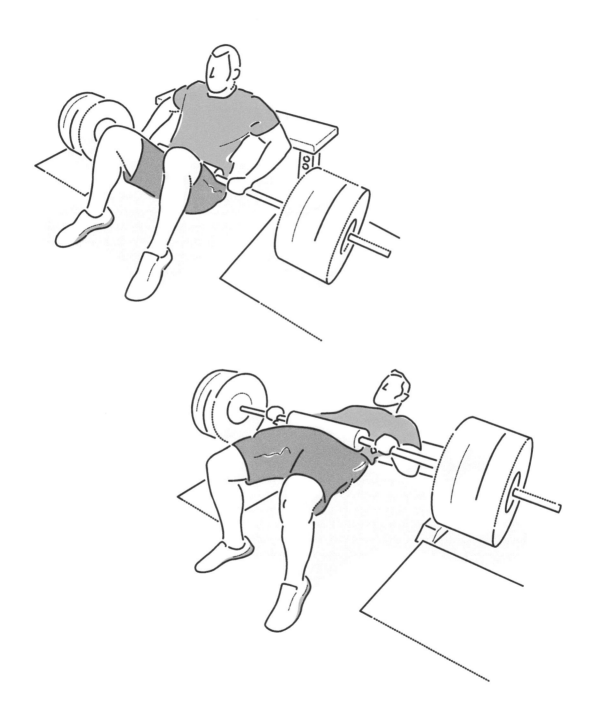

Romanian Deadlift with Barbell

Specific Muscles Involved: Hamstrings, Glutes, Lower Back

The Romanian Deadlift (RDL) with Barbell is one of my favorite exercises! It places more emphasis on the hamstrings than a traditional Deadlift (see page 127). In fact, the RDL is one of the best hamstring exercises you can perform. But be advised: Due to the nature of the exercise, it causes a lot of muscle soreness.

Instructions

The Setup

1. The Romanian Deadlift starts with the barbell in a rack, just above the knees.

2. Standing with feet shoulder-width apart, grab the bar with an overhand grip, brace your core, and lift the bar out of the rack by extending the knees. From there, take a step back. This is the starting position.

The Romanian Deadlift

3. Once in the starting position, brace the core and begin the exercise by hinging at the hips. While hinging, bend forward and push your hips back as the bar slides down your thighs. Maintain a slight bend in the knees.

4. Once the bar is lowered to mid-shin, reverse the movement by driving hips forward and extending the torso back to the starting position.

Practice Makes Perfect

Avoid turning this exercise into a regular Deadlift (see page 127). Maintain only a slight bend in the knees and keep the hips high throughout the entire movement. If you feel the need to bend the knees further, chances are you're using too much weight.

Training Tip

At the top of the range of motion, avoid leaning back. Only go up until your spine is in a neutral position.

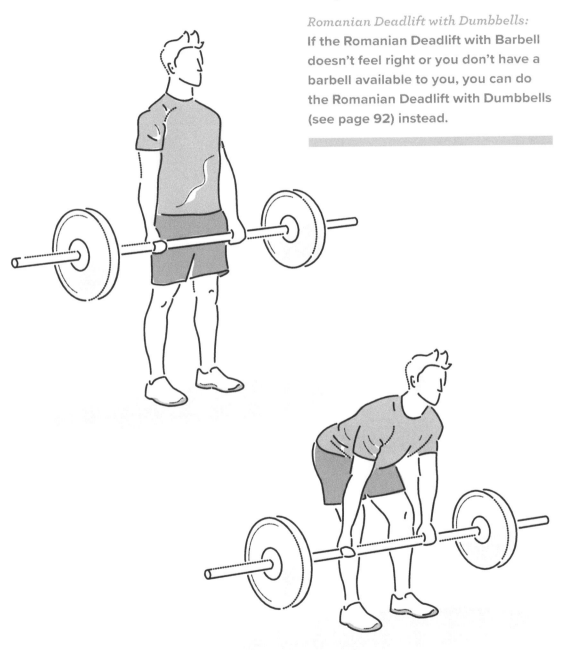

Easy Does It

Romanian Deadlift with Dumbbells:
If the Romanian Deadlift with Barbell doesn't feel right or you don't have a barbell available to you, you can do the Romanian Deadlift with Dumbbells (see page 92) instead.

Bench Press

Specific Muscles Involved: Chest

The Bench Press is probably my all-time favorite exercise. The Bench Press can be a very safe lift if done correctly. But, like any exercise, if done incorrectly it can be problematic. Incorrect form on the bench has most likely caused more shoulder injuries than any other exercise. However, it's also responsible for more upper body muscle growth and strength than any other exercise in existence. So, if we can learn the right technique, this exercise can be very beneficial!

Instructions

The Setup

1. Lie on a flat bench and position yourself so that your eyes are below the racked bar.

2. Before grasping the bar, arch your back, and squeeze together your shoulder blades. Think about trying to hold a pencil in your upper back. This is the most effective way to bench press the most weight, and the safest. Use your legs to help drive your upper back into the bench.

3. Grasp the bar with an even grip that is slightly wider than your shoulders.

4. Lift the bar out of the rack and position it over the chest with the arms fully extended. This is the starting position.

The Bench Press

5. Take a deep breath, brace your core, and lower the bar to touch your chest approximately at the level of the nipples.

6. After a brief pause, push the bar back to the starting position. Focus on pushing the bar up and slightly back toward the rack.

7. Once back at the starting position, hold for one second, then start the next rep.

8. When you are done, place the bar back in the rack.

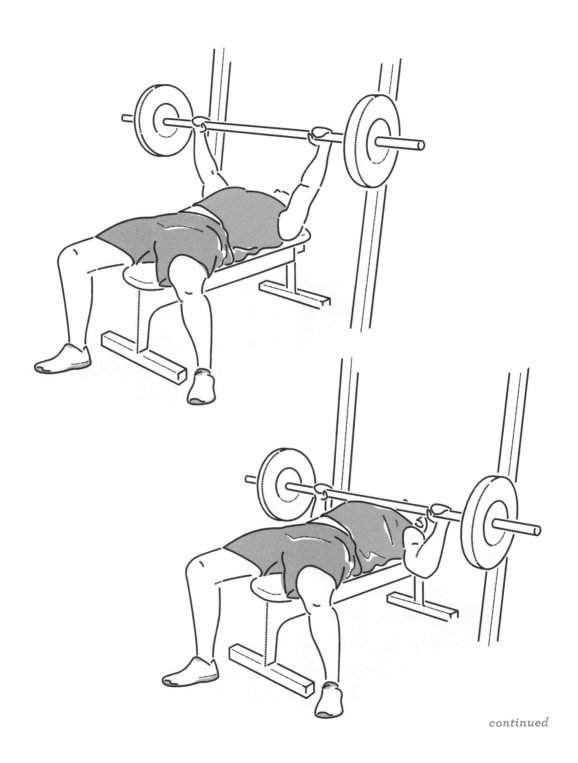

continued

Practice Makes Perfect

A common mistake with this exercise is allowing the butt to come up off the bench during the rep. This can not only lead to lower back pain, but also makes for a less effective Bench Press. The butt can come up for a few different reasons, but the most popular reason is improper direction of leg drive.

Although the Bench Press is an upper body lift, the lower body plays an important role. The more leg drive you can use, the more weight you can press. However, when it comes to leg drive, we want to focus on pushing our toes through the front of our shoes. Tension should be going forward along the surface of the ground, not straight down. Getting this right can keep your butt on the bench and add pounds to the bar.

Training Tip

Where you grip the bar largely depends on personal preference and limb length. Generally speaking, having longer arms will require a wider grip. Play around with different grip widths until you find a position that is comfortable and allows you to lift the most amount of weight.

Easy Does It

Flat Bench Press with Dumbbells: If the barbell Bench Press is too difficult at first, or if you don't have access to a barbell, you can stick with the Flat Bench Press with Dumbbells (see page 98).

Close-Grip Bench Press

Specific Muscles Involved: Chest, Triceps

The Close-Grip Bench Press is a bench variation that works the triceps as much as, if not more than, it does the chest. This is a great exercise to gain muscle and strength in the triceps. Also, due to the extended range of motion and different grip, the Close-Grip Bench Press helps improve the regular Bench Press (see page 134) as well.

Instructions

The Setup

1. Lie back on a flat bench and place the body so that the eyes are below the racked bar.

2. Before grasping the bar, arch your back while squeezing your shoulder blades together. Think about trying to hold a pencil in your upper back. This is not only the most effective way to bench press the most weight, but also it is the safest. Use your legs to help drive your upper back into the bench.

3. Once you're set, grasp the bar with a close grip, slightly closer than shoulder-width.

4. Lift the bar out of the rack and position it over the chest with the arms fully extended. This is the starting position.

The Close-Grip Bench Press

5. Take a deep breath, brace your core, and lower the bar to touch the middle part of the chest. Unlike the regular Bench Press, it's important to keep the elbows tucked in during the entire rep.

6. After a brief pause, push the bar back to the starting position. Focus on pushing the bar up and slightly back toward the rack.

7. Once you are back at the starting position, hold for a second and then start the next rep.

8. When you are done with the prescribed number of reps, place the bar back in the rack.

continued

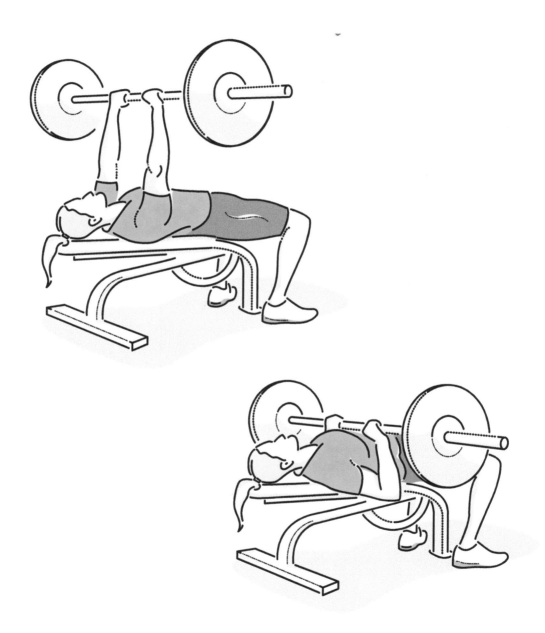

Practice Makes Perfect

A common mistake with the Close-Grip Bench Press is actually gripping the bar too close. Don't take the name too literally. If you grip the bar too close it puts unneeded pressure on the wrists and limits how much weight you can use. Grip the bar slightly closer than shoulder-width to gain maximum benefits from the movement.

Training Tip

Try to set up and execute the lift the same way you would a regular Bench Press. The only tangible difference is the grip width.

Easy Does It

Close-Grip Push-Up: If the Close-Grip Bench Press is too difficult, doing a Close-Grip Push-Up is an excellent bodyweight variation to work the chest and triceps.

Incline Bench Press with Barbell

Specific Muscles Involved: Chest

The barbell Incline Bench Press is an exercise that targets the upper chest. I'm a big fan of the dumbbell version of this exercise, but the barbell offers the ability to handle more weight. The key with the barbell Incline Bench Press is finding a grip width that's comfortable on your shoulders.

Instructions

The Setup

1. Set up an incline bench to an angle between 30 and 45 degrees, or use a fixed-incline Bench Press station. Make sure you adjust the incline bench so that your eyes are directly under the bar. If the bench is too far away or too close to the bar, taking the bar off the rack will be too difficult.

2. Before grasping the bar, start by getting yourself situated in a good position on the bench. Lie on your back with your shoulder blades retracted and feet firmly planted on the floor, and grip the barbell with a slightly wider than shoulder-width grip.

3. To begin, unrack the bar and hold it with your arms straight so that the bar is directly above your upper chest. This is your starting position.

The Incline Bench Press

4. Start the movement by lowering the bar under control until it lightly touches your chest. Hold the bar paused on your chest for one second before pressing the bar back up to the starting position. Repeat for the desired amount of reps.

Practice Makes Perfect

A common issue with the barbell Incline Bench Press is lowering the bar too high or too low. Lower the bar to the mid-chest.

Training Tip

If your gym doesn't have a dedicated barbell Incline Bench Press station, you can create one by putting an adjustable bench in a power rack. If your gym doesn't have an adjustable bench, you can create an incline by stacking a couple of 45-pound plates under one end of a flat bench to prop it up.

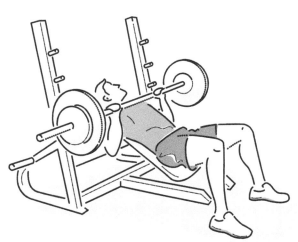

Easy Does It

Incline Bench Press with Dumbbells: Some people experience shoulder pain when performing the barbell Incline Bench Press. If that happens to you, you can stick to the Incline Bench Press with Dumbbells (see page 100).

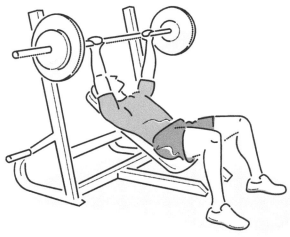

Overhead Press

Specific Muscles Involved: Shoulders

The Overhead Press is the king of shoulder exercises. Nothing will put meat across your entire shoulder area like the Overhead Press will. This is also one of the few shoulder exercises where you can overload with heavy weights. However, this is also an exercise that can cause shoulder injuries if your form is incorrect. Make sure you warm up well and have good technique before adding weight to the bar.

Instructions

The Setup

1. Start with a barbell in a rack at around chest level. Grasp the barbell with an overhand grip, slightly wider than shoulder-width. Position the bar in front of your neck at the collarbone. This is the starting position.

The Overhead Press

2. Take a deep breath, brace your core, flex your glutes, and press the bar upward until your arms are extended overhead. As the bar is being pressed overhead, bring your head and chest forward.

3. Return the bar to the starting position.

Practice Makes Perfect

A common mistake is turning the Overhead Press into what is called a "Push Press." A Push Press uses leg drive to get the barbell overhead, which takes some tension off the shoulders. You want your shoulders to lift the weight overhead, not your legs. To avoid using too much leg drive, maintain a slight knee bend during the movement but limit any lower body movement.

Training Tip

Find a foot position that is comfortable for you. I personally like a narrow, less than shoulder-width stance, but this is not required.

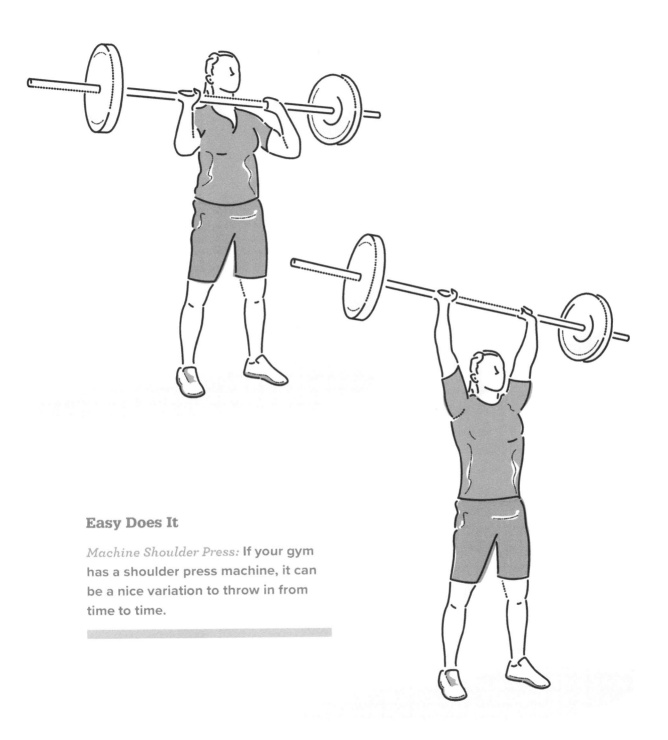

Easy Does It

Machine Shoulder Press: If your gym has a shoulder press machine, it can be a nice variation to throw in from time to time.

Barbell Row

Specific Muscles Involved: Back

There is no denying the benefits of the Barbell Row. It's one of the staple back-building movements. The biggest benefit of the Barbell Row is the fact that you can handle more weight on a Barbell Row than you can on any other row variation.

Instructions

The Setup

1. Stand with the legs slightly bent and shoulder-width apart, grasping the bar with an overhand grip. The hands should be slightly wider than shoulder-width apart.

2. There are a few variations, but for the purpose of this book, lean forward at the waist 45 degrees so that with the arms extended the bar hangs around the knees. This is the starting position.

The Barbell Row

3. Pull the bar toward the torso. Keep the torso rigid. Avoid jerking the torso upward as you pull.

4. Touch the bar to the lower part of the abdomen and lower the bar back to the starting position.

Practice Makes Perfect

The biggest mistake when performing a Barbell Row is using the full body to lift the weight. The goal of this exercise is to build muscle in the upper back and lat regions, not to see how much weight we can throw around. During the movement, keep the torso rigid and the knees slightly bent. Don't allow the back or knee angle to change as you are rowing the barbell up.

Training Tip

If you're feeling this more in your lower back than in your upper back, you're using too much weight.

Easy Does It

Inverted Row: If the Barbell Row is too difficult or causes lower back pain, an alternative is the Inverted Row (see page **68**).

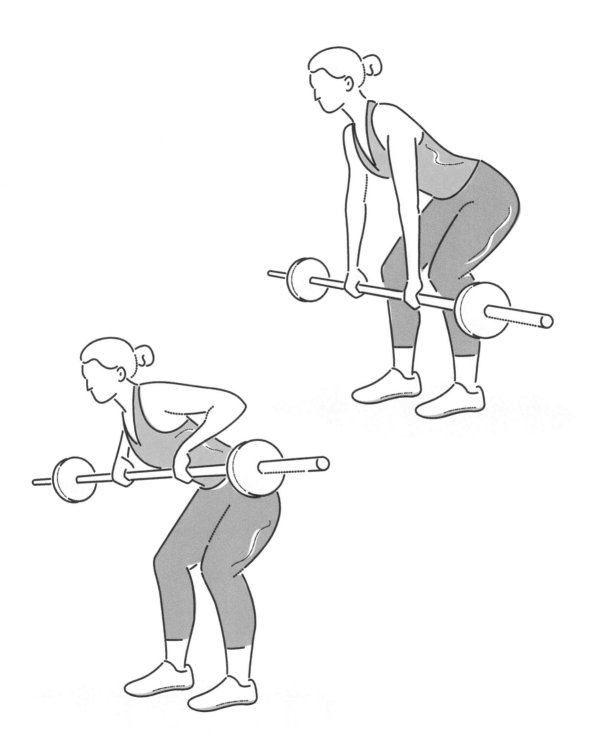

Barbell Shrug

Specific Muscles Involved: Traps

Nothing looks quite as powerful on a physique as big traps. It's one of the first things you notice when a lifter passes you on the street. When it comes to building traps, the Barbell Shrug is the best movement pattern to use. The Barbell Shrug is a very simple exercise with a limited range of motion that allows you to handle a lot of weight.

Instructions

1. Hold a bar in an overhand grip with your hands just outside shoulder-width.

2. Lift your shoulders straight up, making sure to elevate them as high as possible. Hold the top position for one full second before lowering the shoulders back to the starting position.

Practice Makes Perfect

The biggest mistake with the Barbell Shrug is rolling the shoulders. This motion is not only less effective, but also can lead to injury. Simply move your shoulders up and down during the movement.

Training Tip

Since the range of motion is so limited with this exercise, it's important to use as much range of motion as possible. Allow the weights to drop as low as possible at the bottom and raise your shoulders as high as possible at the top.

Easy Does It

If Barbell Shrugs don't feel comfortable, using a pair of dumbbells for Shrugs can put your hands in a more natural position.

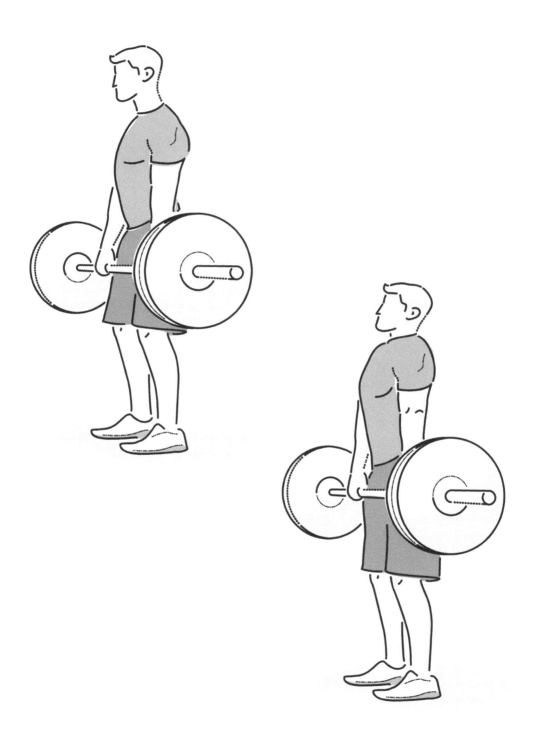

Upright Row with Barbell

Specific Muscles Involved: Traps, Shoulders

The Upright Row is an exercise that has fallen out of favor in recent years. The trouble is, if done incorrectly, the Upright Row can lead to shoulder pain. However, if it is done correctly, it is a great shoulder and trap builder that hits both muscles in a unique movement pattern.

Instructions

1. Start by grasping a barbell using an overhand grip with the palms facing down and hands shoulder-width apart.

2. Standing straight up and with your abs braced, raise the bar up your torso toward your shoulders. Raise the bar until it reaches right under your chin.

3. Hold the top of the range of motion for a second before slowly lowering the weight back to the starting position.

Practice Makes Perfect

During the movement, it is important to lead with the elbows. Your elbows should be higher than your wrists at all times.

Training Tip

A wider grip will incorporate more side delts into the movement.

Easy Does It

Sometimes the Upright Row can cause shoulder pain. If this is the case for you, replace the barbell with dumbbells and perform the same movement.

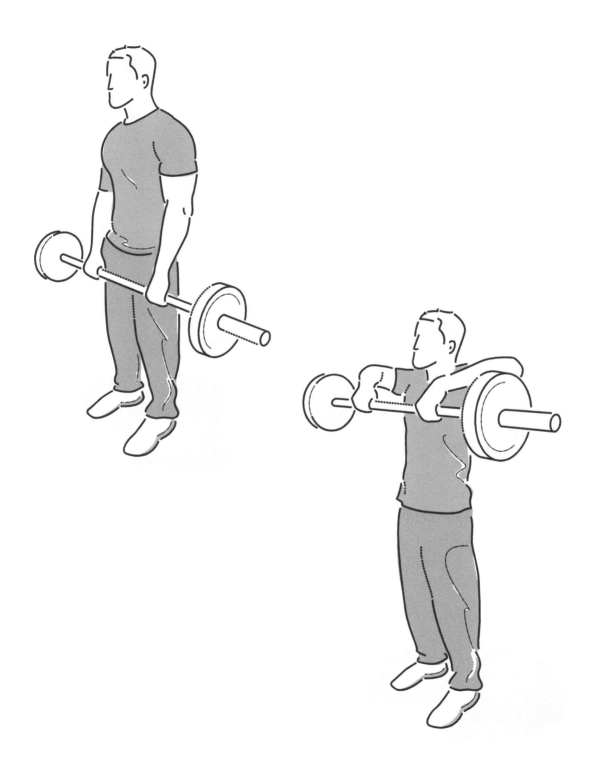

Barbell Curl

Specific Muscles Involved: Biceps

When you think of Curls, you probably think of Barbell Curls. The Barbell Curl is the biceps exercise that will allow you to use the most weight and put the most mass onto your biceps. I probably don't need to sell you any harder on this one.

Instructions

The Setup

1. Stand straight up, grasping the bar with a closed, underhand grip. The grip should be shoulder-width, so the arms touch the sides of your torso. Allow your arms to be fully extended. This is the starting position.

The Barbell Curl

2. Curl the weight until the bar is near the front of the shoulders. Be mindful of your elbow position. Don't let the elbows drift forward during the movement.

3. Once the bar reaches the shoulders, slowly lower the bar back to the starting position.

Practice Makes Perfect

We want to take the lower body out of the movement in this exercise. No body part other than the arms should move while you are curling the weight. Lock your legs and torso in place and prevent any rocking back and forth or arching in the lower back.

Training Tip

The Barbell Curl allows for multiple grips, ranging from narrow to wide. Using different grip widths will provide slightly different results. However, finding a grip that is comfortable on your wrists and elbows is most important.

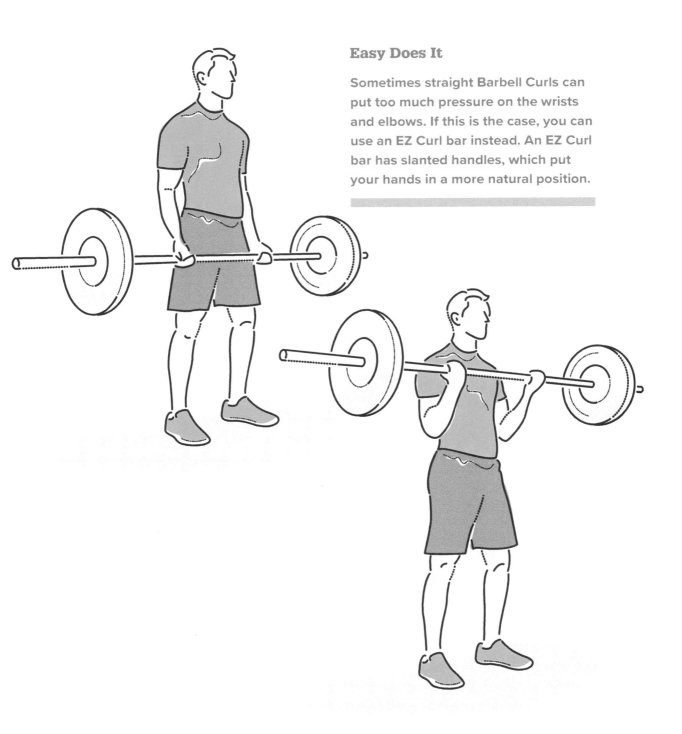

Easy Does It

Sometimes straight Barbell Curls can put too much pressure on the wrists and elbows. If this is the case, you can use an **EZ Curl bar** instead. An **EZ Curl bar** has slanted handles, which put your hands in a more natural position.

Reverse Curl

Specific Muscles Involved: Biceps

The Reverse Curl incorporates the forearms more than any other biceps exercise. Developing the forearms not only helps improve your grip, but also gives you a strong and powerful look.

Instructions

The Setup

1. Stand erect, grasping the bar with an open overhand grip. Your palms should be facing your body. The grip should be shoulder-width so that the arms touch the sides of your torso. Allow your arms to be fully extended. This is the starting position.

The Reverse Curl

2. Curl the weight until the bar is near the front of the shoulders. Be mindful of your elbow position. Don't let the elbows drift forward during the movement.

3. Once the bar reaches the shoulders, slowly lower the bar back to the starting position.

Practice Makes Perfect

Elbow positioning is crucial with the Reverse Curl. You want to keep the elbows locked down for the entire rep. Avoid letting the elbows drift forward or out to the sides.

Training Tip

On the Reverse Curl, we use what's called an open grip. This means you don't wrap your thumb around the bar; instead, your thumb goes on the same side as the rest of your fingers. This helps add extra emphasis to the forearms.

Easy Does It

If the Reverse Curl feels unnatural, you can do the same movement holding dumbbells. The dumbbell variation allows the wrists to move freely, which can be more comfortable.

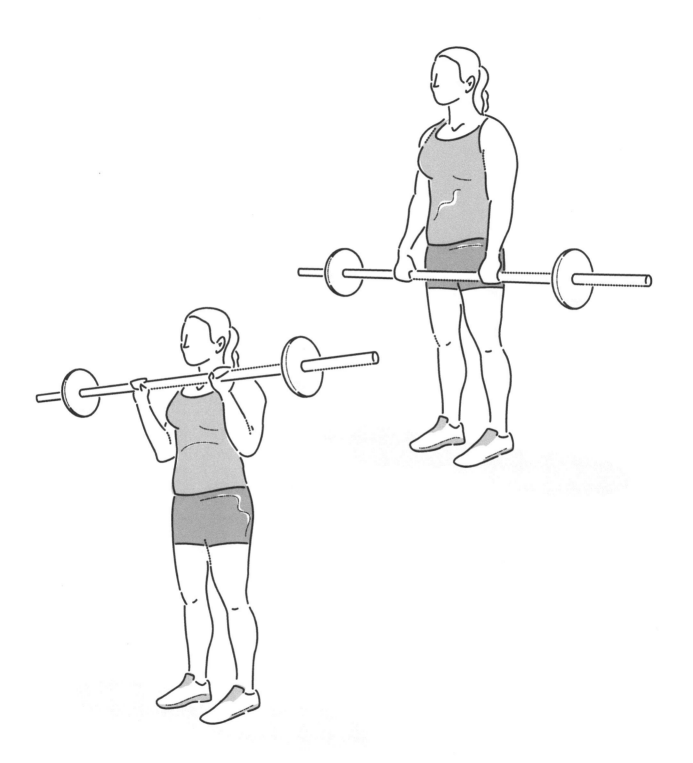

Lying Triceps Extension

Specific Muscles Involved: Triceps

The Lying Triceps Extension, a.k.a. "the Skullcrusher," has been a bodybuilding staple for years. The key is finding the right grip width and range of motion that feels best for you. Some people experience elbow pain if this is done incorrectly, so this is an exercise where you want to pay special attention to technique.

Instructions

The Setup

1. Lie on your back on a bench and grasp a barbell with a closed overhand grip, at about shoulder-width.

2. Position the bar over the chest with the arms locked out at full extension. The elbows should be pointed toward the knees. This is the starting position.

The Lying Triceps Extension

3. Keep your upper arms stationary as the elbows bend, bringing the bar toward your forehead.

4. Keep the wrists stiff and upper arms perpendicular to the floor the duration of the rep.

5. Lower the bar until it almost touches the forehead and return back to the starting position using your triceps.

Practice Makes Perfect

Avoid allowing the elbows to flare out toward the sides. This turns the exercise into a press, which incorporates more chest and less triceps.

Training Tip

You can lower the bar to your face, forehead, or even behind your head. All locations work, so find which area feels best for you and use that.

Easy Does It

Close-Grip Push-Up: A great bodyweight variation for this exercise is a Close-Grip Push-Up (page 139).

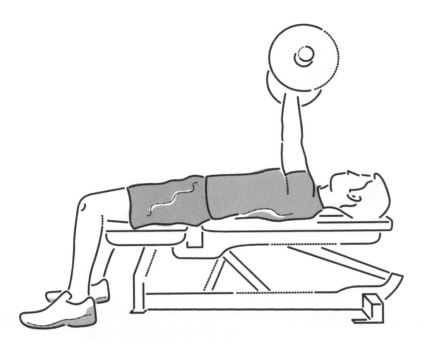

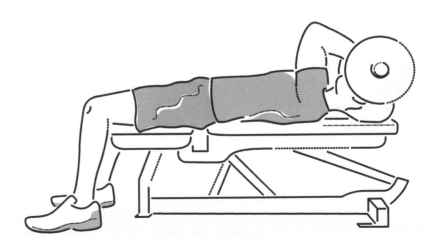

Windshield Wiper

Specific Muscles Involved: Abdominals, Chest, Shoulders

The Windshield Wiper might be the least common exercise in this book. Chances are you won't find many people in your local gym performing this movement. But don't let that fool you; this one is very difficult. It's a lot more than just an abdominal exercise; it targets almost the entire torso, directly or indirectly.

Instructions

1. Lie on your back on the floor holding a lightly loaded barbell directly above your chest in a Bench Press position. Keep both legs extended out straight.

2. To start the movement, while holding the barbell over your chest, lift both legs toward the left plate on the barbell and do your best to touch the plate with your feet.

3. After touching the left weight plate, lower both legs back to the starting position and repeat on the other side. Doing the movement on each side equals one rep.

Practice Makes Perfect

A common mistake with this exercise is overestimating your strength. Don't be afraid to start really light. If you use too much weight, you won't be able to perform the exercise effectively.

Training Tip

Start really light with this exercise. Using just the bar with no weights added is probably the best place to start.

Easy Does It

Broomstick Windshield Wiper: You can perform the movement without holding a barbell. Just hold a broomstick instead. The exercise is performed the exact same way.

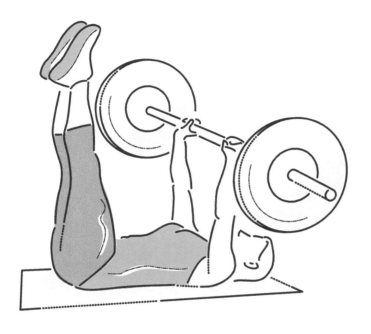

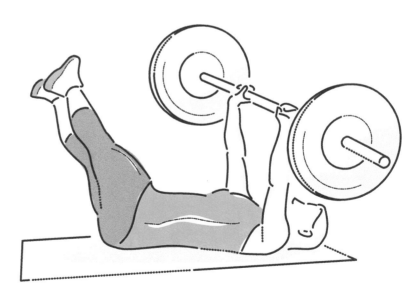

Rollout

Specific Muscles Involved: Abdominals

The Rollout is my personal favorite when it comes to ab exercises. The ab wheel is underused and underappreciated, but there's no doubt it is brutally effective. If your gym doesn't have one, you can pick one up online. It's worth the investment to have in your gym bag. You can also use a barbell with 10-pound plates on each side and do Rollouts with that.

Instructions

The Setup

1. Position yourself in a kneeling position with your knees about hip-width apart and grasp the ab roller with both hands. The ab roller should be on the floor in front of you. This will be your starting position.

The Rollout

2. Slowly roll the ab roller forward, stretching your body into a straight position. Just like in the Plank (see page 86), make sure the movement isn't coming from your spine or from your hips. Maintain a neutral spine throughout the set.

3. Go down as low as you can without any part of your body touching the floor other than your knees and feet.

4. After a pause at the end range of motion, start pulling yourself back with your core to the starting position. Keep your abs tight at all times.

Practice Makes Perfect

This is a tough exercise when done correctly. The biggest mistake people make is allowing their hips to sag. Keep your core tight and your glutes flexed to help keep the torso in a straight line.

Training Tip

If going out to full extension is too hard, start by going only halfway. Slowly over time, work your way up to doing the full range of motion.

Easy Does It

Plank: If the Rollout is too difficult, you can start by getting really proficient at the Plank (see page 86).

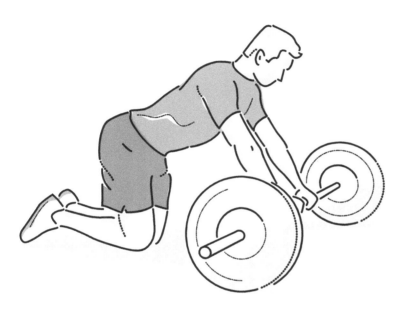

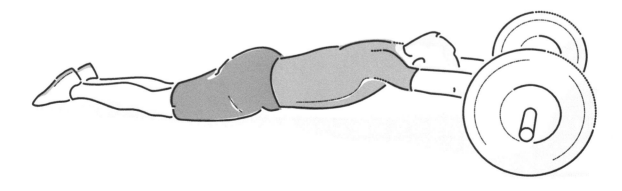

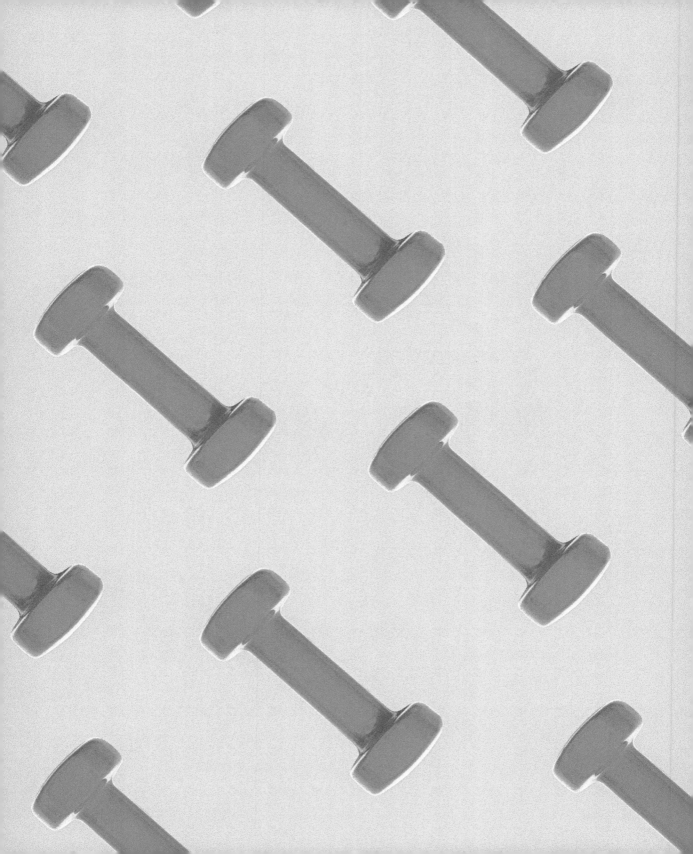

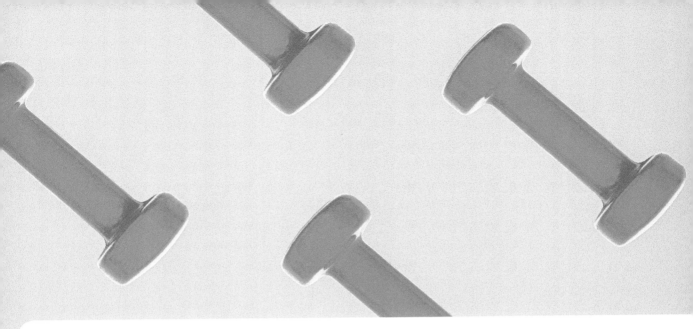

Part Three

THE 12-WEEK PROGRAM

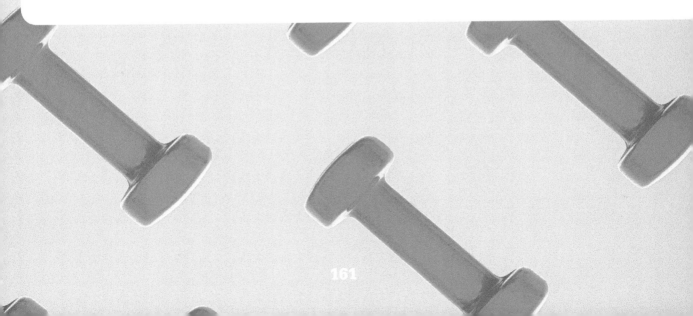

N ow we enter what's arguably the most important section of the book—the program! At the end of the day, I can provide you with all the information in the world, but until you take action, you won't get stronger. Throughout this section, there will be many tips and tricks to help you get the most out of the workouts. If you have any questions about form or technique, you can always refer back to the exercise section and review the illustrations and directions.

The workouts are designed to be completed in 60 to 90 minutes, including the warm-up and cooldown. The first week of each phase will probably be closer to 90 minutes as you get accustomed to the exercises, but each week thereafter should be more efficient as the exercises become more familiar.

To allow for optimal recovery and performance, perform the workouts every other day. As an example, do workout A on Monday, workout B on Wednesday, and workout C on Friday. With this schedule, you could choose to take the weekend off, or start back with workout A on Sunday.

Month One: Bodyweight

Month one is a bodyweight-only program. The biggest benefit to bodyweight exercises is accessibility. These are workouts you can do anywhere and anytime because they require no equipment! If an exercise is too easy or too difficult for the programmed amount of reps, refer back to the exercise section and select a more appropriate option.

WORKOUT A

Warm-Up

Start with 5 minutes of light cardiovascular activity.

Complete 2 rounds, resting about 60 seconds between rounds.

1. Jumping Jacks x 10 reps
2. Leg Swings x 10 reps each side
3. Arm Circles x 10 reps each direction
4. Bird Dog x 5 reps each side
5. Thoracic Bridge x 5 reps each side

Exercises

Complete the reps for exercises 1 to 4 in as few sets as possible, making sure to rest as needed.

1. Air Squat x 60 reps
2. Push-Up x 60 reps
3. Glute Bridge x 60 reps
4. Pull-Up x 30 reps

Complete exercises 5a/b and 6a/b back-to-back with no rest. Rest 1 to 2 minutes between exercises 5a/b and 6a/b.

- 5a. Flexed Arm Hang, 3 sets x 15- to 30-second hold
- 5b. Bicycle Crunch, 3 sets x 15 to 20 reps each side
- 6a. Handstand Push-Up, 3 sets x 6 to 8 reps
- 6b. Single-Leg Calf Raise, 3 sets x 15 to 30 reps

Cooldown

1. Couch Stretch, 2 sets x 15- to 30-second hold each side
2. Hurdle Stretch, 2 sets x 15- to 30-second hold each side
3. Lat Stretch, 2 sets x 15- to 30-second hold each side
4. Dead Hang, 2 sets x 10 to 15 seconds
5. Foam Roll IT Band, 1 set x 30 seconds on each side
6. Foam Roll Lats, 1 set x 30 seconds on each side
7. Foam Roll Adductors, 1 set x 30 seconds on each side
8. Foam Roll Upper Back, 1 set x 30 seconds

Strength Tip:

Keep track of all of your workouts in a training journal. You can use an app or go old school with a composition notebook. This will help you stay organized and optimize your workouts. Keep track of sets, reps, how you felt during the workout, how long the workout took to complete, etc.

WORKOUT B

If an exercise is too easy or too difficult for the programmed amount of reps, refer back to the exercise section and select a more appropriate option.

Warm-Up

Start with 5 minutes of light cardiovascular activity.

Complete 2 rounds, resting about 60 seconds between rounds.

1. Mountain Climbers x 10 reps each side
2. Leg Swings x 10 reps each side
3. Scapular Push-Up x 10 reps
4. Fire Hydrant x 5 reps each side
5. Thoracic Bridge x 5 reps each side

Exercises

Complete the reps for exercises 1 to 4 in as few sets as possible, making sure to rest as needed.

1. Air Squat x 30 reps
2. Push-Up x 30 reps
3. Glute Bridge x 30 reps
4. Pull-Up x 15 reps

Complete exercises 5a/b and 6a/b back-to-back with no rest. Rest 1 to 2 minutes between exercises 5a/b and 6a/b.

- 5a. Inverted Row, 3 sets x 10 to 12 reps
- 5b. Plank, 3 sets x 30- to 60-second hold
- 6a. Bench Dips, 3 sets x 10 to 12 reps
- 6b. Superman, 3 sets x 10 to 12 reps

Cooldown

1. Couch Stretch, 2 sets x 15- to 30-second hold each side
2. Hurdle Stretch, 2 sets x 15- to 30-second hold each side
3. Lat Stretch, 2 sets x 15- to 30-second hold each side
4. Dead Hang, 2 sets x 10 to 15 seconds
5. Foam Roll IT Band, 1 set x 30 seconds on each side
6. Foam Roll Lats, 1 set x 30 seconds on each side
7. Foam Roll Adductors, 1 set x 30 seconds on each side
8. Foam Roll Upper Back, 1 set x 30 seconds

WORKOUT C

If an exercise is too easy or too difficult for the programmed amount of reps, refer back to the exercise section and select a more appropriate option.

Warm-Up

Start with 5 minutes of light cardiovascular activity.

Complete 2 rounds, resting about 60 seconds between rounds.

1. Jumping Jacks x 10 reps
2. Leg Swings x 10 reps each side
3. Arm Circles x 10 reps each direction
4. Bird Dog x 5 reps each side
5. Thoracic Bridge x 5 reps each side

Exercises

Complete the reps for exercises 1 to 4 in as few sets as possible, making sure to rest as needed.

1. Air Squat x 80 reps
2. Push-Up x 80 reps
3. Glute Bridge x 80 reps
4. Pull-Up x 40 reps

Complete exercises 5a/b and 6a/b back-to-back with no rest. Rest 1 to 2 minutes between exercises 5a/b and 6a/b.

- 5a. Y-W-T Isohold, 3 sets x 10- to 20-second hold in each position
- 5b. Hanging Leg Raise, 3 sets x 10 to 12 reps
- 6a. Parallel Bar Dips, 3 sets x 10 to 12 reps
- 6b. Cossack Squat, 3 sets x 8 to 10 reps each side

Cooldown

1. Couch Stretch, 2 sets x 15- to 30-second hold each side
2. Hurdle Stretch, 2 sets x 15- to 30-second hold each side
3. Lat Stretch, 2 sets x 15- to 30-second hold each side
4. Dead Hang, 2 sets x 10 to 15 seconds
5. Foam Roll IT Band, 1 set x 30 seconds on each side
6. Foam Roll Lats, 1 set x 30 seconds on each side
7. Foam Roll Adductors, 1 set x 30 seconds on each side
8. Foam Roll Upper Back, 1 set x 30 seconds

Month Two: Bodyweight + Dumbbell

This month, we're adding in dumbbells. Dumbbells offer the unique opportunity to work both sides of the body independently while adding a stabilization challenge. If an exercise is too easy or too difficult for the programmed amount of reps, refer back to the exercise section and select a more appropriate option.

WORKOUT A

Warm-Up

Start with 5 minutes of light cardiovascular activity.

Complete 2 rounds, resting about 60 seconds between rounds.

1. Jumping Jacks x 10 reps
2. Leg Swings x 10 reps each side
3. Arm Circles x 10 reps each direction
4. Bird Dog x 5 reps each side
5. Thoracic Bridge x 5 reps each side

Exercises

Rest 2 to 3 minutes between sets.

1. Goblet Squat, 3 sets x 7 reps
2. Flat Bench Press with Dumbbells, 3 sets x 7 reps
3. Romanian Deadlift with Dumbbells, 3 sets x 7 reps
4. Dumbbell Row, 3 sets x 7 reps

Complete exercises 5a/b and 6a/b back-to-back with no rest. Rest 1 to 2 minutes between exercises 5a/b and 6a/b.

- 5a. Side Raise, 3 sets x 8 to 10 reps
- 5b. Dumbbell Pullover, 3 sets x 8 to 10 reps
- 6a. Single-Leg Calf Raise with Dumbbells, 3 sets x 8 to 10 reps
- 6b. Weighted Sit-Up, 3 sets x 8 to 10 reps

Cooldown

1. Couch Stretch, 2 sets x 15- to 30-second hold each side
2. Hurdle Stretch, 2 sets x 15- to 30-second hold each side
3. Lat Stretch, 2 sets x 15- to 30-second hold each side
4. Dead Hang, 2 sets x 10 to 15 seconds
5. Foam Roll IT Band, 1 set x 30 seconds on each side
6. Foam Roll Lats, 1 set x 30 seconds on each side
7. Foam Roll Adductors, 1 set x 30 seconds on each side
8. Foam Roll Upper Back, 1 set x 30 seconds

WORKOUT B

Warm-Up

Start with 5 minutes of light cardiovascular activity.

Complete 2 rounds, resting about 60 seconds between rounds.

1. Mountain Climbers x 10 reps each side
2. Leg Swings x 10 reps each side
3. Scapular Push-Up x 10 reps
4. Fire Hydrant x 5 reps each side
5. Thoracic Bridge x 5 reps each side

Exercises

Rest 2 to 3 minutes between sets.

1. Air Squat, 3 sets x 10 reps
2. Standing Shoulder Press, 3 sets x 10 reps
3. Weighted Lunges, 3 sets x 10 reps
4. Pull-Ups, 3 sets x 10 reps

Complete exercises 5a/b and 6a/b back-to-back with no rest. Rest 1 to 2 minutes between exercises 5a/b and 6a/b.

- 5a. Hammer Curl, 3 sets x 8 to 10 reps
- 5b. Triceps Kickbacks, 3 sets x 8 to 10 reps
- 6a. Push-Up, 3 sets x 8 to 10 reps
- 6b. Side Bend, 3 sets x 8 to 10 reps each side

Cooldown

1. Couch Stretch, 2 sets x 15- to 30-second hold each side
2. Hurdle Stretch, 2 sets x 15- to 30-second hold each side
3. Lat Stretch, 2 sets x 15- to 30-second hold each side
4. Dead Hang, 2 sets x 10 to 15 seconds
5. Foam Roll IT Band, 1 set x 30 seconds on each side
6. Foam Roll Lats, 1 set x 30 seconds on each side
7. Foam Roll Adductors, 1 set x 30 seconds on each side
8. Foam Roll Upper Back, 1 set x 30 seconds

WORKOUT C

Warm-Up

Start with 5 minutes of light cardiovascular activity.

Complete 2 rounds, resting about 60 seconds between rounds.

1. Jumping Jacks x 10 reps
2. Leg Swings x 10 reps each side
3. Arm Circles x 10 reps each direction
4. Bird Dog x 5 reps each side
5. Thoracic Bridge x 5 reps each side

Exercises

Rest 2 to 3 minutes between sets.

1. Goblet Squat, 3 sets x 5 reps
2. Incline Bench Press with Dumbbells, 3 sets x 5 reps
3. Romanian Deadlift with Dumbbells, 3 sets x 5 reps
4. Dumbbell Row, 3 sets x 5 reps

Complete exercises 5a/b and 6a/b back-to-back with no rest. Rest 1 to 2 minutes between exercises 5a/b and 6a/b.

- 5a. Alternating Curl, 3 sets x 8 to 10 reps
- 5b. Overhead Triceps Extension with Dumbbells, 3 sets x 8 to 10 reps
- 6a. Single-Leg Calf Raise with Dumbbells, 3 sets x 8 to 10 reps
- 6b. Plank, 3 sets x 30- to 60-second hold

Cooldown

1. Couch Stretch, 2 sets x 15- to 30-second hold each side
2. Hurdle Stretch, 2 sets x 15- to 30-second hold each side
3. Lat Stretch, 2 sets x 15- to 30-second hold each side
4. Dead Hang, 2 sets x 10 to 15 seconds
5. Foam Roll IT Band, 1 set x 30 seconds on each side
6. Foam Roll Lats, 1 set x 30 seconds on each side
7. Foam Roll Adductors, 1 set x 30 seconds on each side
8. Foam Roll Upper Back, 1 set x 30 seconds

Strength Tip:

If you are struggling with technique, take a video of yourself lifting. Sometimes watching yourself on video can help identify where your technique needs correcting.

Month Three: Bodyweight + Dumbbell + Barbell

Finally, in month three we'll incorporate the gold standard of strength modalities: the barbell. A barbell offers the best way to lift the most weight, which makes it perfect for strength training. If an exercise is too easy or too difficult for the programmed amount of reps, refer back to the exercise section and select a more appropriate option.

WORKOUT A

Warm-Up

Start with 5 minutes of light cardiovascular activity.

Complete 2 rounds, resting about 60 seconds between rounds.

1. Jumping Jacks x 10 reps
2. Leg Swings x 10 reps each side
3. Arm Circles x 10 reps each direction
4. Bird Dog x 5 reps each side
5. Thoracic Bridge x 5 reps each side

Exercises

Rest 2 to 3 minutes between sets.

1. Back Squat, 3 sets x 5 reps
2. Bench Press, 3 sets x 5 reps
3. Romanian Deadlift with Barbell, 3 sets x 5 reps
4. Barbell Row, 3 sets x 5 reps

Complete exercises 5a/b and 6a/b back-to-back with no rest. Rest 1 to 2 minutes between exercises 5a/b and 6a/b.

- 5a. Incline Bench Press with Barbell, 3 sets x 6 to 8 reps
- 5b. Upright Row with Barbell, 3 sets x 6 to 8 reps
- 6a. Barbell Curl, 3 sets x 6 to 8 reps
- 6b. Plank, 3 sets x 30- to 60-second hold

Cooldown

1. Couch Stretch, 2 sets x 15- to 30-second hold each side
2. Hurdle Stretch, 2 sets x 15- to 30-second hold each side
3. Lat Stretch, 2 sets x 15- to 30-second hold each side
4. Dead Hang, 2 sets x 10 to 15 seconds
5. Foam Roll IT Band, 1 set x 30 seconds on each side
6. Foam Roll Lats, 1 set x 30 seconds on each side
7. Foam Roll Adductors, 1 set x 30 seconds on each side
8. Foam Roll Upper Back, 1 set x 30 seconds

Strength Tip:

Now that you're using barbells, make sure you have a spotter when you're doing heavy sets. If you're not working out with a training partner, don't be afraid to ask someone to assist you. Safety is important!

WORKOUT B

Warm-Up

Start with 5 minutes of light cardiovascular activity.

Complete 2 rounds, resting about 60 seconds between rounds.

1. Mountain Climbers x 10 reps each side
2. Leg Swings x 10 reps each side
3. Scapular Push-Up x 10 reps
4. Fire Hydrant x 5 reps each side
5. Thoracic Bridge x 5 reps each side

Exercises

Rest 2 to 3 minutes between sets.

1. Goblet Squat, 3 sets x 7 reps
2. Overhead Press, 3 sets x 7 reps
3. Hip Thrust, 3 sets x 7 reps
4. Pull-Ups, 3 sets x 7 reps

Complete exercises 5a/b and 6a/b back-to-back with no rest. Rest 1 to 2 minutes between exercises 5a/b and 6a/b.

- 5a. Close-Grip Bench Press, 3 sets x 6 to 8 reps
- 5b. Side Raise, 3 sets x 6 to 8 reps
- 6a. Reverse Curl, 3 sets x 6 to 8 reps
- 6b. Windshield Wiper, 3 sets x 6 to 12 reps each side

Cooldown

1. Couch Stretch, 2 sets x 15- to 30-second hold each side
2. Hurdle Stretch, 2 sets x 15- to 30-second hold each side
3. Lat Stretch, 2 sets x 15- to 30-second hold each side
4. Dead Hang, 2 sets x 10 to 15 seconds
5. Foam Roll IT Band, 1 set x 30 seconds on each side
6. Foam Roll Lats, 1 set x 30 seconds on each side
7. Foam Roll Adductors, 1 set x 30 seconds on each side
8. Foam Roll Upper Back, 1 set x 30 seconds

WORKOUT C

Warm-Up

Start with 5 minutes of light cardiovascular activity.

Complete 2 rounds, resting about 60 seconds between rounds.

1. Jumping Jacks x 10 reps
2. Leg Swings x 10 reps each side
3. Arm Circles x 10 reps each direction
4. Bird Dog x 5 reps each side
5. Thoracic Bridge x 5 reps each side

Exercises

Rest 2 to 3 minutes between sets.

1. Back Squat, 3 sets x 3 reps
2. Bench Press, 3 sets x 3 reps
3. Deadlift, 3 sets x 3 reps
4. Barbell Row, 3 sets x 5 reps

Complete exercises 5a/b and 6a/b back-to-back with no rest. Rest 1 to 2 minutes between exercises 5a/b and 6a/b.

- 5a. Lying Triceps Extension, 3 sets x 6 to 8 reps
- 5b. Barbell Shrug, 3 sets x 6 to 8 reps
- 6a. Single-Leg Calf Raise with Dumbbell, 3 sets x 6 to 8 reps
- 6b. Rollout, 3 sets x 6 to 12 reps

Cooldown

1. Couch Stretch, 2 sets x 15- to 30-second hold each side
2. Hurdle Stretch, 2 sets x 15- to 30-second hold each side
3. Lat Stretch, 2 sets x 15- to 30-second hold each side
4. Dead Hang, 2 sets x 10 to 15 seconds
5. Foam Roll IT Band, 1 set x 30 seconds on each side
6. Foam Roll Lats, 1 set x 30 seconds on each side
7. Foam Roll Adductors, 1 set x 30 seconds on each side
8. Foam Roll Upper Back, 1 set x 30 seconds

You did it! Hopefully, you were able to gain strength both physically and mentally over the course of the last 12 weeks. Ultimately, it's what you do after these 12 weeks that will be most important. Fitness is a game of consistency. For lasting results, continue showing up. Take advantage of the opportunity to learn and expand your training knowledge through the resources at the end of this book. You're in control now. Good luck!

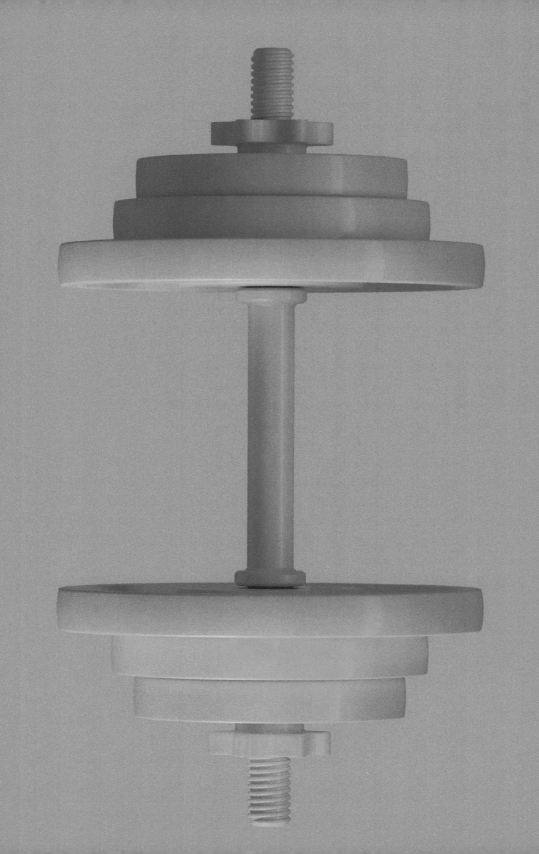

Resources

Here's a list of resources to help you continue progressing on your strength training journey.

Websites

Hunt Fitness: *kylehuntfitness.com*. I provide hundreds of free resources, including articles, podcasts, interviews, and videos here for you to learn more about weightlifting. I also offer one-on-one online coaching if you want to take the next step in your fitness journey.

The Absolute Strength Podcast: *kylehuntfitness.com/category/podcast*. On the podcast, I answer questions and interview some of the biggest names in the fitness industry. Find it on my website or iTunes, Stitcher, Google Play, YouTube, and Spotify.

Rogue Fitness: *roguefitness.com*. Rogue Fitness, the industry leader in American-made strength and conditioning equipment, is the place for almost everything you could ever need for workouts, including squat racks, barbells, knee sleeves, belts, shoes, and more.

Books

Delavier, Frédéric. *Strength Training Anatomy*. Champaign, IL: Human Kinetics, 2006. *Strength Training Anatomy* is a great book if you want to dive deeper into human musculature and anatomy.

Hunt, Kyle. *Bodybuilding for Beginners*. Emeryville, CA: Rockridge Press, 2019. One of my other books, *Bodybuilding for Beginners*, primarily focuses on building muscle. It would be a great complement to the 12-week strength building program in *Strength Training for Beginners*.

Starrett, Kelly, and Glen Cordoza. *Becoming a Supple Leopard: The Ultimate Guide to Resolving Pain, Preventing Injury, and Optimizing Athletic Performance, 2nd Edition*. Las Vegas: Victory Belt Publishing, 2015. This is an excellent book to read to learn more about mobility and soft tissue work. In order to make progress, you have to keep your body healthy, and this book can help you do just that.

Index

Acknowledgments

The acknowledgements section is one of the hardest for me to write. I always feel like I'm going to leave someone out. The truth is, nothing great is ever accomplished without a lot of help. Over the past year, I dove headfirst into becoming a writer. It has quickly become one of the most fun and rewarding parts of my career. I want to give a huge thank-you to Callisto Media and Rockridge Press for continuing to give me the opportunity to write. I look forward to more projects in the future. Second, I have to give my entire family a shout-out. Thank you for picking up the slack for me while I got singularly focused on writing. I know I probably don't say it enough, but I appreciate you! Lastly, I have to recognize all of the clients I have had the opportunity to coach over the years. Without all of you, I wouldn't be where I am today.

About the Author

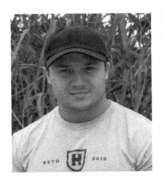

Kyle Hunt is a competitive powerlifter, coach, author, and owner of Hunt Fitness, a highly sought-after online fitness and nutrition coaching business. Kyle specializes in building workout and nutrition programs customized to each of his client's goals. He has worked with hundreds of individuals, including bodybuilders, physique athletes, powerlifters, wrestlers, and clients from all walks of life aiming to perform or look their best. Kyle has a Bachelor of Science degree in exercise science from Fredonia State University and is a certified fitness trainer and fitness nutrition specialist.